Registered Health Information Administrator (RHIA) Exam Preparation

Seventh Edition

Patricia Shaw,
EdD, RHIA, FAHIMA
and
Darcy Carter,
DHSc, MHA, RHIA
Editors

AHIMA
PRESS

ISBN: **978-1-58426-575-7**

AHIMA Product No.: AB106016

AHIMA Staff:
Chelsea Brotherton, MA, Assistant Editor
Megan Grennan, Senior Production Development Editor
Elizabeth Ranno, Vice President of Product and Planning
Caitlin Wilson, Project Editor
Pamela Woolf, Director of Publications

Cover image: ©9comeback, iStockphoto.com

For more information, including updates, about AHIMA Press publications, visit http://www.ahima.org/education/press.

American Health Information Management Association
233 North Michigan Avenue, 21st Floor
Chicago, Illinois 60601-5809
ahima.org

Contents

About the Editors

Patricia Shaw, EdD, RHIA, FAHIMA, holds a doctorate and master's degree in education. Dr. Shaw has been on the faculty of Weber State University since 1991 where she teaches in the health information management and health services administration programs. She has primary teaching responsibility for the quality and performance improvement, coding, reimbursement, and data management curriculum in those programs. Prior to accepting a position at Weber State University, Dr. Shaw managed hospital health information services departments and was a nosologist for 3M Health Information Systems. Dr. Shaw is also co-author of *Quality and Performance Improvement in Healthcare: Theory, Practice, and Management* published by AHIMA.

Darcy Carter, DHSc, MHA, RHIA, earned her doctorate degree in health science with an emphasis in leadership and organizational behavior and her master's degree in healthcare administration. She is on the faculty in the health information management and technology programs at Weber State University, where she teaches courses in coding, reimbursement, and database management. Dr. Carter is also co-author of *Quality and Performance Improvement in Healthcare: Theory, Practice, and Management* published by AHIMA.

Acknowledgments

The authors would like to acknowledge Lauree Handlon, MS, RHIA, CCS, CPC-H, FAHIMA for her contributions to this text.

About the AHIMA RHIA Exam

Job opportunities for Registered Health Information Administrators (RHIAs) exist in multiple settings throughout the healthcare industry. These include the continuum of care delivery organizations, including hospitals, multispecialty clinics and physician practices, long-term care, mental health, and other ambulatory care settings. The profession has seen significant expansion in nonpatient care settings, with careers in managed care and insurance companies, software vendors, consulting services, government agencies, education, and pharmaceutical companies.

Working as a critical link between care providers, payers, and patients, an RHIA:

- Is an expert in managing patient health information and medical records, administering computer information systems, collecting and analyzing patient data, and using classification systems and medical terminologies.
- Possesses comprehensive knowledge of medical, administrative, ethical, and legal requirements and standards related to healthcare delivery and the privacy of protected patient information.
- Manages people and operational units, participates in administrative committees, and prepares budgets.
- Interacts with all levels of an organization—clinical, financial, administrative, and information systems—that employ patient data in decision-making and everyday operations.

The National Commission for Certifying Agencies (NCCA) has granted accreditation to AHIMA's RHIA certification program. This accomplishment establishes AHIMA as the industry leader in accredited health information and informatics management (HIIM) certification programs, and advances AHIMA's organizational mission of positioning AHIMA members and certificants as recognized leaders in advancing professional practice and standards in HIIM.

The Commission on Certification for Health Informatics and Information Management (CCHIIM) manages and sets the strategic direction for the certifications. Pearson Vue is the exclusive provider of AHIMA certification exams. To see sample questions and images of the new exam format, visit the AHIMA website. For more detailed information, including eligibility requirements, visit http://www.ahima.org/certification/RHIA.

Exam Competency Statements

A certification exam is based on an explicit set of competencies. These competencies have been determined through a job analysis study conducted of practitioners. The competencies are subdivided into domains and tasks, as listed here. Each domain is allocated a predefined number of questions at specific cognitive levels to make up the exam. The RHIA exam tests only content pertaining to the following competencies.

Domain 1: Data Content, Structure, and Standards (18–22% of exam)

- ***Classification Systems***
  - Code diagnosis and procedures according to established guidelines.
- ***Health Record Content and Documentation***
  - Ensure accuracy and integrity of health data and health record documentation (paper or electronic).
  - Manage the contents of the legal health record (structured and unstructured).
  - Manage the retention and destruction of the legal health record.

- ***Data Governance***
  - Maintain data in accordance with regulatory requirements.
  - Develop and maintain organizational policies, procedures, and guidelines for management of health information.
- ***Data Management and Secondary Data Sources***
  - Manage health data elements or data sets.
  - Assist in the maintenance of the data dictionary and data models for database design.
  - Manage and maintain databases (for example, data migration, updates).

Domain 2: Information Protection: Access, Disclosure, Archival, Privacy, and Security (18–27% of exam)

- ***Health Law***
  - Maintain healthcare privacy and security training programs.
  - Enforce and monitor organizational compliance with healthcare information laws, regulations, and standards (for example, audit, report, or inform).
- ***Data Privacy, Confidentiality, and Security***
  - Design policies and implement privacy practices to safeguard protected health information (PHI).
  - Design policies and implement security practices to safeguard PHI.
  - Investigate and resolve healthcare privacy and security issues or breaches.
- ***Release of Information***
  - Manage access, disclosure, and use of PHI to ensure confidentiality.
  - Develop policies and procedures for uses and disclosures or redisclosures of PHI.

Domain 3: Informatics, Analytics, and Data Use (22–26% of exam)

- ***Health Information Technologies***
  - Implement and manage use of, and access to, technology applications.
  - Evaluate and recommend clinical, administrative, and specialty service applications (for example, financial systems, electronic record, clinical coding).
- ***Information Management Strategic Planning***
  - Present data for organizational use (for example, summarize, synthesize, and condense information).
- ***Analytics and Decision Support***
  - Filter or interpret information for the end customer.
  - Analyze and present information to organizational stakeholders.
  - Use data mining techniques to query and report from databases.
- ***Healthcare Statistics***
  - Calculate healthcare statistics for organizational stakeholders.
  - Critically analyze and interpret healthcare statistics for organizational stakeholders (for example, CMI).
- ***Research Methods***
  - Identify appropriate data sources for research.
- ***Consumer Informatics***
  - Identify or respond to the information needs of internal and external healthcare customers.
  - Provide support for enduser portals and personal health records.

- ***Health Information Exchange***
    - Apply data and functional standards to achieve interoperability of healthcare information systems.
    - Manage the health information exchange process entity-wide.
- ***Information Integrity and Data Quality***
    - Apply data/record storage principles and techniques associated with the medium (for example, paper-based, hybrid, electronic).
    - Manage master person index (for example, patient record integration, customer/client relationship management).
    - Manage merge process for duplicates and other errors entity-wide (for example, validate data sources).

Domain 4: Revenue Management (12–16% of exam)

- ***Revenue Cycle and Reimbursement***
    - Manage the use of clinical data required in reimbursement systems and prospective payment systems (PPS).
    - Optimize reimbursement through management of the revenue cycle (for example, chargemaster maintenance, DNFB, and AR days).
- ***Regulatory***
    - Prepare for accreditation and licensing processes (for example, Joint Commission, Det Norske Veritas [DNV], Medicare, state regulators).
    - Process audit requests (for example, RACs or other payors, chart review).
    - Perform audits (for example, chart review, POC).
- ***Coding***
    - Manage or validate coding accuracy.
- ***Fraud Surveillance***
    - Participate in investigating incidences of medical identity theft.
- ***Clinical Documentation Improvement***
    - Query physicians for appropriate documentation to support reimbursement.
    - Educate and train clinical staff regarding supporting documentation requirements.

Domain 5: Leadership (12–16% of exam)

- ***Leadership Roles***
    - Develop, motivate, and support work teams or individuals (for example, coaching).
    - Organize and facilitate meetings.
    - Advocate for department, organization, or profession.
- ***Change Management***
    - Participate in the implementation of new processes (for example, systems, EHRs, CAC).
    - Support changes in the organization (for example, culture changes, HIM consolidations, outsourcing)
- ***Work Design and Process Improvement***
    - Establish and monitor productivity standards
    - Analyze and design workflow processes
    - Participate in the development and monitoring of process improvement plans

- ***Human Resources Management***
    - Perform human resource management activities (for example, recruiting staff, creating job descriptions, resolving personnel issues)
- ***Training and Development***
    - Conduct training and educational activities (for example HIM systems, coding, medical and institutional terminology, documentation and regulatory requirements)
- ***Strategic and Organizational Management***
    - Monitor industry trends and organizational needs to anticipate changes.
    - Determine resource needs by performing analyses (for example, cost-benefit, business planning).
    - Assist with preparation of capital budget.
- ***Financial Management***
    - Assist in preparation and management of operating and personnel budgets.
    - Assist in the analysis and reporting on budget variances.
- ***Ethics***
    - Adhere to the AHIMA code of ethics.
- ***Project Management***
    - Utilize appropriate project management methodologies.
- ***Vendor or Contract Management***
    - Evaluate and manage contracts (for example, vendor, contract personnel, maintenance).
- ***Enterprise Information Management***
    - Develop and support strategic and operational plans for entity-wide health information management.

AHIMA RHIA Exam Specifications

The AHIMA RHIA exam is made up of 180 multiple choice questions. The computer will monitor the time you spend on the exam. A clock in the upper-right corner of the screen will indicate the time remaining to complete the exam. The exam will terminate at the allotted four-hour time limit.

During the exam, candidates are provided all of the appropriate information to answer a question on the exam. Therefore, commonly-used hospital statistical formulas are provided if a question requires calculations that go beyond basic rates and percentages. These formulas are also listed in the Resources section of this book. A calculator will also be available during the exam.

The *International Classification of Diseases, Tenth Revision, Clinical Modification* (ICD-10-CM), *International Classification of Diseases, Tenth Revision, Procedure Coding System* (ICD-10-PCS), *Current Procedural Terminology* (CPT), and *Healthcare Common Procedure Coding System* (HCPCS) coding concepts will be tested on the AHIMA RHIA exam. However, coding books will not be needed to take the exam. All necessary information needed to answer a coding question will be included as part of the question. This will include the code, narrative, and other information that may need to be reproduced from the code books. For more AHIMA RHIA exam information, visit the AHIMA website.

How to Use This Book

The RHIA practice questions and exams in this book and on the accompanying website test knowledge of content pertaining to the RHIA competencies published by AHIMA.

The multiple choice practice questions and exams in this book and on its companion website are presented in a similar format to those that might be found on the AHIMA RHIA exam. The book contains 460 multiple choice practice questions and two practice exams (with 180 questions each). Because each question is organized by and identified with one of the five RHIA domains, you will be able to determine whether you need knowledge or skill building in particular areas of the exam domains. Each answer includes a rationale and reference. Sources for question answers listed in the answer key will help you build your knowledge and skills in specific domains.

To effectively use this book, work through all of the exam questions first. This will help you identify areas in which you may need further preparation. For the questions that you answer incorrectly, read the associated references to help refresh your knowledge. After going through the exam questions, answer the practice questions. Again, for the questions that you answer incorrectly, refresh your knowledge by reading the associated references.

Retake the practice questions and exams as many times as you like. To help build your knowledge and skills, you should review the references provided for all questions that you answered incorrectly.

The accompanying website for *RHIA Exam Preparation*, Seventh Edition (listed on the front, inside cover of this book), contains 820 questions—the same 460 practice questions and answers and two practice exams and answers printed in the book. Each of the self-scoring exams can be run in practice mode, which allows you to work at your own pace, or exam mode, which simulates the 4-hour timed exam experience. The practice questions and simulated exams online can be set to be presented in random order, or you may choose to go through the questions in sequential order by domain. You may also choose to practice or test your skills on specific domains. For example, if you would like to build your skills in domain 3, you may choose only domain 3 questions for a given practice session.

The website also includes a glossary of electronic flash cards for 3,500+ health information management-related terms and definitions as well as a listing of commonly used formulas that are available to test takers during the AHIMA RHIA exam.

Test Taking Tips

The best way to prepare for the AHIMA RHIA Certification Exam is to study the material you have learned over the course of your health information administrator educational program. As it is difficult to remember everything you have learned over the course of the program, it is important to review the information. This is best done using this textbook and the tips found above in "How to Use This Book." Carefully review the information in the Commission on Certification for Health Informatics and Information Management Candidate Guide located in the accompanying website for this book (listed on the front, inside cover). You will want to prepare yourself mentally, physically, and emotionally to succeed.

Other tips while studying:

- Be sure to get enough sleep.
- Eat a healthy, well balanced diet.
- Stay hydrated.
- Take a break.
- Get some exercise.
- Do not try to memorize everything; work at understanding.
- Use tricks to remember the material, like using an acronym or other type of word or visual association.
- Try to eliminate other stressors, if possible.
- Take a practice exam in the four-hour time frame you will have for the exam.
- If you do not know where the testing center is located, visit it before the day of the exam. This will help you avoid getting lost or being late for your exam.
- Review the information on your Authorization to Test (ATT) letter.

Exam Day Tips

- Get enough sleep in the days leading up to the exam.
- Wear clothes that you are comfortable in and dress in layers so that you can remove or add a sweater based on the temperature of the room.
- Eat a good breakfast and give yourself enough time to get ready to leave so you are not rushed.
- Arrive at the testing center 30 minutes prior to your exam time with your required identification.
- You will have four hours to complete the exam. Do not obsess over the clock in the room, but do budget your time. This should allow you to answer each question and review any questions you may want to revisit. Time management will be an important part of taking the exam.
- Be sure to read each question carefully. Do not automatically assume you know the answer to a question without first reading the entire question and each answer choice carefully. After reviewing each answer, choose the best answer.
- Skip questions that you do not know the answer to or that are difficult and come back to them. You may find something in another question that helps you to recall information you need to answer a question you skipped. Be sure to manage your time well while you do this.
- Be sure to answer every test question. A "guess" is better than not taking the opportunity to answer a question. But, do so after carefully reviewing the question and the possible answers. After eliminating answers you know are incorrect, make the best selection. A true guess will give you a one-in-four chance of getting a question correct.
- Remember to relax as much as possible and BREATHE. You can do this!

PRACTICE EXAM 1

Domain 1 Data Content, Structure, and Standards

1. Mildred Smith was admitted to a nursing facility with the following information: "Patient is being admitted for Organic Brain Syndrome." Underneath the diagnosis her medical information was listed along with a summary of the care already provided. This information is documented on the:

   a. Admitting physical evaluation record
   b. Patient's rights acknowledgment form
   c. Release of information form
   d. Transfer record

2. A 65-year-old white male was admitted to the hospital on 1/15 complaining of abdominal pain. The attending physician requested an upper GI series and laboratory evaluation of CBC and UA. The x-ray revealed possible cholelithiasis, and the UA showed an increased white blood cell count. The patient was taken to surgery for an exploratory laparoscopy, and a ruptured appendix was discovered. The chief complaint was:

   a. Abdominal pain
   b. Cholelithiasis
   c. Exploratory laparoscopy
   d. Ruptured appendix

3. Mrs. Smith's admitting data indicates that her birth date is March 21, 1948. On the discharge summary, Mrs. Smith's birth date is recorded as July 21, 1948. Which data quality element is missing from Mrs. Smith's health record?

   a. Data accuracy
   b. Data consistency
   c. Data accessibility
   d. Data comprehensiveness

4. Data that have been grouped into meaningful categories according to a classification system are referred to as this type of data:

   a. Research
   b. Reference
   c. Coded
   d. Demographic

5. Which of the following is an acceptable means of authenticating a record entry?

   a. The physician's assistant signs for the physician.
   b. The HIM clerk stamps entries with the physician's signature stamp.
   c. The charge nurse signs the physician's name.
   d. The physician personally signs the entry.

6. All documentation entered in the medical record relating to the patient's diagnosis and treatment are considered this type of data:

   a. Clinical
   b. Financial
   c. Identification
   d. Secondary

7. In a long-term care setting, these are problem-oriented frameworks for additional patient assessment based on problem identification items (triggered conditions):

   a. Resident Assessment Protocols (RAPs)
   b. Resident Assessment Instrument (RAI)
   c. Utilization Guidelines (UG)
   d. Minimum Data Sets (MDS)

8. Conducting an inventory of the facility's records, determining the format and location of record storage, assigning each record a time period for preservation, and destroying records that are no longer needed are all components of a:

   a. Case mix index
   b. Master patient index
   c. Health record matrix
   d. Retention program

9. What is the principal function of health records?

   a. Determine appropriate resource allocation
   b. Serve as the repository of clinical documentation relevant to the care of individual patients
   c. Provide information for performance improvement activities
   d. Support billing and reimbursement processes

10. What type of information makes it easy for hospitals to compare and combine the contents of multiple patient health records?

    a. Administrative information
    b. Demographic information
    c. Progress notes
    d. Uniform data sets

11. When defining the legal health record in a healthcare entity, it is best practice to establish a policy statement of the legal health record as well as a:

    a. Case mix index
    b. Master patient index
    c. Health record matrix
    d. Retention schedule

12. Which of the following materials are required elements in an emergency care record?

    a. Patient's instructions at discharge and a complete medical history
    b. Time and means of the patient's arrival, treatment rendered, and instructions at discharge
    c. Time and means of the patient's arrival, patient's complete medical history, and instructions at discharge
    d. Treatment rendered, instructions at discharge, and the patient's complete medical history

13. In ICD-10-PCS, what value is used if there is a character that does not apply to a given code?

a. X

b. –

c. 0

d. Z

14. Which of the following is the unique identifier in the relational database patient table?

Patient Table			
Patient #	**Patient Last Name**	**Patient First Name**	**Date of Birth**
021234	Smith	Donna	03/21/1944
022366	Jones	Donna	04/09/1960
034457	Smith	Mary	08/21/1977

a. Patient last name

b. Patient last and first name

c. Patient date of birth

d. Patient number

15. Which of the following is used by a long-term care facility to gather information about specific health status factors and includes information about specific risk factors in the resident's care?

a. Case management

b. Minimum Data Set

c. Outcomes and assessment information set

d. Core measure abstracting

16. Mr. Smith was admitted to University Hospital by Dr. Collins. Mr. Smith's hospital bill will be paid by Blue Cross Insurance. Upon discharge from the hospital, who owns the health record of Mr. Smith?

a. Mr. Smith

b. Blue Cross

c. University Hospital

d. Dr. Collins

17. Documenting the full depth and breadth of data use in a healthcare entity requires:

a. Identifying all of the data consumers

b. Identifying the needs of data consumers

c. Understanding all of the functionality requirements

d. Performing a gap analysis

18. Which part of the problem-oriented health record is used by many facilities that have adopted the whole problem-oriented format?

a. The problem list as an index

b. The initial plan

c. The SOAP form of progress notes

d. The database

19. A 45-year-old woman is admitted for blood loss anemia due to dysfunctional uterine bleeding.

D25.9	Leiomyoma of uterus, unspecified
D50.0	Iron deficiency anemia secondary to blood loss (chronic)
D62	Acute posthemorrhagic anemia
N93.8	Other specified abnormal uterine and vaginal bleeding

a. D50.0, N93.8

b. D62, N93.8

c. N93.8, D50.0

d. D50.0, D25.9

20. The insured party's member identification number is an example of this type of data:

a. Demographic data

b. Clinical data

c. Certification data

d. Financial data

21. What is the data model that is most widely used to illustrate a relational database structure?

a. Entity-relationship diagram (ERD)

b. Object model

c. Relational model

d. Unified medical language system (UMLS)

22. A patient arrived via ambulance to the emergency department following a motor vehicle accident. The patient sustained a fracture of the ankle, 3.0 cm superficial laceration of the left arm, 5.0 cm laceration of the scalp with exposure of the fascia, and a concussion. The patient received the following procedures: x-ray of the ankle that showed a bimalleolar ankle fracture requiring closed manipulative reduction and simple suturing of the arm laceration and layer closure of the scalp. Provide CPT codes for the procedures done in the emergency department for the facility bill.

12002	Simple repair of superficial wounds of scalp, neck, axillae, external genitalia, trunk and/or extremities (including hands and feet); 2.6 cm to 7.5 cm
12004	Simple repair of superficial wounds of scalp, neck, axillae, external genitalia, trunk and/or extremities (including hands and feet); 7.6 cm to 12.5 cm
12032	Repair, intermediate, wounds of scalp, axillae, trunk and/or extremities (excluding hands and feet); 2.6 cm to 7.5 cm
27810	Closed treatment of bimalleolar ankle fracture (e.g., lateral and medial malleoli, or lateral and posterior malleoli, or medial and posterior malleoli); with manipulation
27818	Closed treatment of trimalleolar ankle fracture; with manipulation
-58	Staged or related procedure or service by the same physician or other qualified health care professional during the postoperative period
-59	Distinct procedural service

a. 27810, 12032

b. 27818, 12004, 12032-58

c. 27810, 12032, 12002-59

d. 27810, 12004

23. Which of the following is an example of a M:M relationship?

a. Patients to hospital admissions
b. Patients to consulting physicians
c. Patients to hospital health records
d. Primary care physician to patients

24. A patient has a malunion of an intertrochanteric fracture of the right hip that is treated with a proximal femoral osteotomy by incision. What is the correct ICD-10-PCS code for this procedure?

Section	Body System	Root Operation	Body Part	Approach	Device	Qualifier
Medical and Surgical	Lower Bones	Excision	Upper Femur, Right	Open	No Device	No Qualifier
0	Q	B	6	0	Z	Z

Section	Body System	Root Operation	Body Part	Approach	Device	Qualifier
Medical and Surgical	Lower Bones	Division	Upper Femur, Right	Open	No Device	No Qualifier
0	Q	8	6	0	Z	Z

Section	Body System	Root Operation	Body Part	Approach	Device	Qualifier
Medical and Surgical	Lower Joints	Excision	Hip Joint, Right	Open	No Device	No Qualifier
0	S	B	9	0	Z	Z

Section	Body System	Root Operation	Body Part	Approach	Device	Qualifier
Medical and Surgical	Lower Joints	Release	Hip Joint, Right	Open	No Device	No Qualifier
0	S	N	9	0	Z	Z

a. 0QB60ZZ
b. 0Q860ZZ
c. 0SB90ZZ
d. 0SN90ZZ

25. Borrowing record entries from another source as well as representing or displaying past documentation as current are examples of a potential breach of:

    a. Identification and demographic integrity
    b. Authorship integrity
    c. Statistical integrity
    d. Auditing integrity

26. The process by which a person or entity who authored an EHR entry or document seeks to validate that they are responsible for the data contained within it is called:

    a. Endorsement
    b. Confirmation
    c. Authentication
    d. Consent

27. The primary responsibility of a coder is to:

    a. Ensure timely processing of coded data
    b. Ensure accuracy of coded data
    c. Avoid claims rejections by third-party payers
    d. Ensure maximum reimbursement for the facility

28. Documentation including the date of action, method of action, description of the disposed record series of numbers or items, service dates, a statement that the records were eliminated in the normal course of business, and the signatures of the individuals supervising and witnessing the process must be included in this:

    a. Authorization
    b. Certificate of destruction
    c. Informed consent
    d. Continuity of care record

29. Anywhere Hospital has mandated that the Social Security number will be displayed in the XXX-XX-XXXX format for their patients. This is an example of the use of a:

    a. Wildcard
    b. Mask
    c. Truncation
    d. Data definition

30. Using the information in these partial attribute lists for the PATIENT, VISIT, and CLINIC columns in a relational database, the attribute PATIENT_MRN is listed in both the PATIENT Entity Attributes and the VISIT Entity Attributes, and CLINIC_ID is listed in both the VISIT Entity Attributes and the CLINIC Entity Attributes. What does the attribute PATIENT_MRN represent?

PATIENT Entity Attributes

PATIENT_MRN (PK)
PATIENT_LNAME
PATIENT_FNAME
PATIENT_MNAME
PATIENT_STREET
PATIENT_CITY . . .
PATIENT_STATE
PATIENT_ZIPCODE
PATIENT_PHONE
PATIENT_DOB
. . .

VISIT Entity Attributes

VISIT_ID (PK)
VISIT_DATE
VISIT_REASON
PATIENT_MRN (FK)
CLINIC_ID (FK)

CLINIC Entity Attributes

CLINIC_ID (PK)
CLINIC_NAME
CLINIC_STREET
CLINIC_CITY
CLINIC_STATE
CLINIC_ZIPCODE
CLINIC_PHONE
CLINIC_FAX
. . .

a. It is the foreign key in PATIENT and the primary key in VISIT.
b. It is the primary key in PATIENT and the foreign key in VISIT.
c. It is the primary key in both PATIENT and VISIT.
d. It is the foreign key in both PATIENT and VISIT.

31. Decision making and authority over data-related matters is known as

a. Data management
b. Data administration
c. Data governance
d. Data modeling

32. A data element name is considered which of the following?

a. Master data
b. Metadata
c. Structured data
d. Unstructured data

33. A patient is admitted with right diabetic cataract, and extracapsular cataract extraction with simultaneous insertion of intraocular lens.

E11.36	Type 2 diabetes mellitus with diabetic cataract
E11.9	Type 2 diabetes mellitus without complications
H25.9	Unspecified age-related cataract
H26.9	Unspecified cataract

Section	Body System	Root Operation	Body Part	Approach	Device	Qualifier
Medical and Surgical	Eye System	Extraction	Lens, Right	Percutaneous	No Device	No Qualifier
0	8	D	J	3	Z	Z

Section	Body System	Root Operation	Body Part	Approach	Device	Qualifier
Medical and Surgical	Eye System	Replacement	Lens, Right	Percutaneous	Synthetic Substitute	No Qualifier
0	8	R	J	3	J	Z

a. H25.9, E11.36, 08DJ3ZZ

b. E11.36, 08RJ3JZ

c. E11.9, E11.36, H26.9, 08DJ3ZZ

d. E25.9, E11.9, 08RJ3JZ

34. The data elements in a patient's automated laboratory result are examples of:

a. Unstructured data

b. Free-text data

c. Financial data

d. Structured data

35. Abbreviations can be a source of patient safety issues due to misinterpretation and miscommunication. Abbreviations in the health record:

a. Are not permitted by Joint Commission standards

b. Should have only one meaning

c. Enhance patient safety

d. Are critical to an electronic health record system

36. Why could it be difficult for a healthcare entity to respond to pulling an entire, legal health record together for an authorized request for information?

a. It can exist in separate and multiple paper-based or electronic systems.

b. The record is incomplete.

c. Numerous physicians have not given consent to release the record.

d. Risk management will not allow the legal health record to be released.

37. Data mapping is used to harmonize data sets or code sets. The code or data set from which the map originates is the:

a. Source
b. Target
c. Equivalent group
d. Solution

38. Data that are collected on large populations of individuals and stored in databases are referred to as:

a. Statistics
b. Accession data
c. Aggregate data
d. Standards

39. Notes written by physicians and other practitioners as well as dictated and transcribed reports are examples of:

a. Standardized data
b. Codified data
c. Aggregate data
d. Unstructured clinical information

40. A significant challenge when handling hybrid records is complicated by the fact that:

a. Patients will continue to request paper records
b. Providers will continue to demand paper records
c. The requirements, regulations, and constraints of EHRs and paper records must be met
d. Only paper records can be used for legal purposes

41. According to Joint Commission Accreditation Standards, which document must be placed in the patient's record before a surgical procedure may be performed?

a. Admission record
b. Physician's order
c. Report of history and physical examination
d. Discharge summary

Domain 2 *Information Protection: Access, Disclosure, Archival, Privacy, and Security*

42. The legal health record for disclosure consists of:

a. Any and all protected health information data collected or used by a healthcare entity when delivering care
b. Only the protected health information requested by an attorney for a legal proceeding
c. The data, documents, reports, and information that comprise the formal business records of any healthcare entity that are to be utilized during legal proceedings
d. All of the data and information included in the HIPAA Designated Record Set

43. What does an audit trail check for?

a. Loss of data

b. Presence of a virus

c. Successful completion of a backup

d. Unauthorized access to a system

44. A clinic has a contract with the city government to perform all new employee physicals and work injury evaluations. Is it appropriate that a patient's family history of cancer be reported to the employer?

a. No, because this information is considered PHI

b. No, unless the cancer diagnosis is still active

c. Yes, because the employer has the right to access all information on its employees

d. Yes, unless the employer has allowed for such exclusion

45. An outpatient laboratory routinely mails the results of health screening exams to its patients. The lab has received numerous complaints from patients who have received another patient's health information. Even though multiple complaints have been received, no change in process has occurred because the error rate is low in comparison to the volume of mail that is processed daily for the lab. How should the Privacy Officer for this healthcare entity respond to this situation?

a. Determine why the lab results are being sent to incorrect patients and train the laboratory staff on the HIPAA Privacy Rule

b. Fire the responsible employees

c. Do nothing, as these types of errors occur in every healthcare entity

d. Retrain the entire hospital entity because these types of errors could result in a huge fine from the Office of Inspector General

46. Anywhere Hospital's coding staff will be working remotely. The entity wants to ensure that they are complying with the HIPAA Security Rule. What type of network uses a private tunnel through the Internet as a transport medium that will allow the transmission of ePHI to occur between the coder and the facility securely?

a. Intranet

b. Local area network

c. Virtual private network

d. Wide area network

47. Mary Smith has gone to her doctor to discuss her current medical condition. What is the legal term that best describes the type of communication that has occurred between Mary and her physician?

a. Closed communication

b. Open communication

c. Private communication

d. Privileged communication

48. An individual designated as an inpatient coder may have access to an electronic medical record in order to code the record. Under what access security mechanism is the coder allowed access to the system?

a. Context-based
b. Role-based
c. Situation-based
d. User-based

49. Which of the following statements about a firewall is ***false***?

a. It is a system or combination of systems that supports an access control policy between two networks.
b. The most common place to find a firewall is between the healthcare entity's internal network and the Internet.
c. Firewalls are effective for preventing all types of attacks on a healthcare system.
d. A firewall can limit internal users from accessing various portions of the Internet.

50. A dietary department donated its old microcomputer to a school. Some old patient data were still on the microcomputer. What controls would have minimized this security breach?

a. Access controls
b. Device and media controls
c. Facility access controls
d. Workstation controls

51. The Privacy Rule generally requires documentation related to its requirements to be retained:

a. 3 years
b. 5 years
c. 6 years
d. 10 years

52. Mrs. Davis is preparing to undergo hernia repair surgery at Deaconess Hospital. Select the best statement of the following options.

a. An employee from the hospital's surgery department should obtain Mrs. Davis' informed consent.
b. The surgeon should obtain Mrs. Davis' informed consent.
c. It does not matter who obtains Mrs. Davis' informed consent as long as it is documented in her medical record.
d. Informed consent is not necessary because this is not major surgery.

53. Which legal doctrine was established by the *Darling v. Charleston Community Hospital* case of 1965?

a. Hospital–physician negligence
b. Clinical negligence
c. Physician–patient negligence
d. Corporate negligence

54. Which national database was created to collect information on the legal actions (both civil and criminal) taken against licensed healthcare providers?

a. Healthcare Insurance Data Bank

b. Medicare Protection Database

c. National Practitioner Data Bank

d. Healthcare Safety Database

55. Sally Mitchell was treated for kidney stones at Graham Hospital last year. She now wants to review her medical record in person. She has requested to review it by herself in a closed room.

a. Failure to accommodate her wishes will be a violation under the HIPAA Privacy Rule.

b. Sally owns the information in her record, so she must be granted her request.

c. Sally's request does not have to be granted because the hospital is responsible for the integrity of the medical record.

d. Patients should never be given access to their actual medical records.

56. The legal term used to describe when a patient has the right to maintain control over certain personal information is referred to as:

a. Access

b. Confidentiality

c. Privacy

d. Security

57. Who has the legal right to refuse treatment? (Choose all that apply.)

1. Juanita who is 98 years old and of sound mind.
2. Christopher who is 10 years old and of sound mind.
3. Jane who is 35, incompetent, and did not express her treatment wishes prior to becoming incompetent.
4. Linda who is 35, incompetent, and created a living will prior to becoming incompetent stating that she did not wish to be kept alive by artificial means.
5. William who is a 35-year-old born with mental retardation and has the mental capacity of a 12-year-old.

a. 1 and 2

b. 1 and 3

c. 1 and 4

d. 4 and 5

58. Linda Wallace is being admitted to the hospital. She is presented with a Notice of Privacy Practices. In the Notice, it is explained that her PHI will be used and disclosed for treatment, payment, and operations (TPO) purposes. Linda states that she does not want her PHI used for those purposes. Of the options listed here, what is the best course of action?

a. The hospital must honor her wishes and not use her PHI for TPO.

b. The hospital may decline to treat Linda because of her refusal.

c. The hospital is not required to honor her wishes in this situation, as the Notice of Privacy Practices is informational only.

d. The hospital is not required to honor her wishes for treatment purposes but must honor them for payment and operations purposes.

59. When a patient collapses upon arrival at the entrance to an emergency department, what type of treatment authorization is in effect?

a. Emergency consent

b. Expressed consent

c. Informed consent

d. Implied consent

60. Jack Mitchell, a patient in Ross Hospital, is being treated for gallstones. He has not opted out of the facility directory. Callers who request information about him may be given:

a. No information due to the highly sensitive nature of his illness

b. Admission date and location in the facility

c. General condition and acknowledgment of admission

d. Location in the facility and diagnosis

61. What type of access safeguard is more people-focused in nature?

a. Technical

b. Administrative

c. Physical

d. Addressable

62. The federal law that directed the Secretary of Health and Human Services (HHS) to develop healthcare standards governing electronic data interchange and data security is the:

a. Medicare Act

b. Prospective Payment Act

c. Health Insurance Portability and Accountability Act

d. Social Security Act

63. Medical information loses PHI status and is no longer protected by the HIPAA Privacy Rule when it:

a. Is oral communication

b. Is deidentified

c. Is used for TPO

d. Is individually identifiable

64. The Workforce Security Standard has all of the following addressable implementation standards ***except***:

a. Authorization and supervision
b. Workforce clearance procedures
c. Termination procedures
d. Concept supervision

65. Dr. Smith, a member of the medical staff, asks to see the medical records of his adult daughter who was hospitalized in your institution for a tonsillectomy at age 16. The daughter is now 25. Dr. Jones was the patient's physician. Of the options listed here, what is the best course of action?

a. Allow Dr. Smith to see the records because he was the daughter's guardian at the time of the tonsillectomy.
b. Call the hospital administrator for authorization to release the record to Dr. Smith since he is on the medical staff.
c. Inform Dr. Smith that he cannot access his daughter's health record without her signed authorization allowing him access to the record.
d. Refer Dr. Smith to Dr. Jones and release the record if Dr. Jones agrees.

66. St. Joseph's Hospital has a psychiatric service on the sixth floor. A 31-year-old male came to the HIM department and requested to see a copy of his health record. He told the clerk he was a patient of Dr. Schmidt, a psychiatrist, and had been on the sixth floor of St. Joseph's for the last two months. These records are not psychotherapy notes. The best course of action for you to take as the HIM director is:

a. Prohibit the patient from accessing his record as it contains psychiatric diagnoses that may greatly upset him.
b. Allow the patient to access his record.
c. Allow the patient to access his record if, after contacting his physician, his physician does not feel it will be harmful to the patient.
d. Deny access because HIPAA prevents patients from reviewing their psychiatric records.

67. You are a member of the hospital's Health Information Management Committee. The committee has created a HIPAA-compliant authorization form. Which of the following items does the Privacy Rule require for the form?

a. Signature of the patient's attending physician
b. Identification of the patient's next of kin
c. Identification of the person or entity authorized to receive PHI
d. Patient's insurance information

68. Which of the following is an identifier under the Privacy Rule?

a. Gender
b. Vehicle license plate
c. Blood pressure reading
d. Temperature

69. A hospital health information department receives a subpoena duces tecum for records of a former patient. When the health record professional goes to retrieve the patient's medical records, it is discovered that the records being subpoenaed have been purged in accordance with the state retention laws. In this situation, how should the HIM department respond to the subpoena?

a. Inform defense and plaintiff lawyers that the records no longer exist
b. Submit a certification of destruction in response to the subpoena
c. Refuse the subpoena since no records exist
d. Contact the clerk of the court and explain the situation

70. An HIM professional violates privacy protection under the HIPAA Privacy Rule when he or she releases ________ without specific authorization from the patient(s) or patient representative(s).

a. A list of newborns to the local newspaper for publication in the birth announcements section
b. Data about cancer patients to the state health department cancer surveillance program
c. Birth information to the country registrar
d. Information about patients with sexually transmitted infections to the county health department

71. What is the implication regarding the confidentiality of incident reports in a legal proceeding when a staff member documents in the health record that an incident report was completed about a specific incident?

a. There is no impact.
b. The person making the entry in the health record may not be called as a witness in trial.
c. The incident report likely becomes discoverable because it is mentioned in a discoverable document.
d. The incident report cannot be discovered even though it is mentioned in a discoverable document.

72. This federal agency is charged with responsibility for the oversight and enforcement of the HIPAA privacy regulations.

a. The Office of the National Coordinator for Health Information Technology
b. The Centers for Medicare and Medicaid Services
c. The HHS Office of Civil Rights
d. The HHS Office of the Inspector General

73. The Kids' Foundation, a foundation related to Children's Hospital, is mailing fundraising information to the families of all patients who have been treated at Children's in the past three years. Based on the facts given:

a. Children's Hospital violated the Privacy Rule by giving information to the foundation.
b. Children's Hospital must have notified the patients or patients' guardians of this disclosure in the Notice of Privacy Practices.
c. The Kids' Foundation cannot solicit donations from patients' families under any circumstances.
d. The Kids' Foundation must request authorization from each patient or patient guardian to mail fundraising information out to their families.

74. An audit trail is a good tool for which one of the following?

a. Holding an individual patient accountable for actions
b. Reconstructing electronic events
c. Defending the corporation against an IRS audit
d. Stopping attacks from the intranet to the Internet

75. Sometimes federal and state health information privacy laws and regulations are in conflict. When this is the case one law must take precedence. For health information privacy this is determined as follows:

    a. The federal law always takes precedence
    b. The state law always takes precedence
    c. The law that gives the consumer greater rights with respect to their PHI takes precedence
    d. The facility can choose to follow either the state or federal law

76. A hospital employee destroyed a health record so that its contents—which would be damaging to the employee—could not be used at trial. In legal terms, the employee's action constitutes:

    a. Mutilation
    b. Destruction
    c. Spoliation
    d. Spoilage

77. A breach occurs when unsecured protected health information is accessed or released. The Secretary of HHS and local media must be notified if this threshold of patient records breached has been met or exceeded.

    a. 1,000
    b. 500
    c. 100
    d. 10,000

78. The Security Rule leaves the methods for conducting the security risk analysis to the discretion of the healthcare entity. The first consideration for a healthcare facility should be:

    a. Its own characteristics and environment
    b. The potential threats and vulnerabilities
    c. The level of risk
    d. An assessment of current security measures

79. Addressable Security Rule implementation specifications:

    a. Should be implemented unless a healthcare entity determines that the specification is not reasonable and appropriate and documents their reasoning
    b. Are not optional; the healthcare entity must implement them as stated in the regulation
    c. Are required if legal counsel determines this to be true and they do not conflict with state law
    d. Are only required to be read by healthcare entities; they do not have to be implemented

80. Employees, volunteers, trainees, and other persons performing functions on behalf of covered entities and business associates, whether paid or not, are considered to be:

    a. Consultants
    b. Workforce
    c. Immune from prosecution under HIPAA
    d. Vendors

81. Although an addressable implementation specification, this reduces or prevents access and viewing of ePHI.

a. Data management technology

b. Encryption

c. Decryption

d. Anonymization of all data

82. The concept of legal hold requires:

a. Special, tracked handling of patient records involved in litigation to ensure no changes can be made

b. Attorneys for healthcare entities to stop all activity with records involved in litigation

c. All records involved in litigation to be printed and held in a locked cabinet

d. To not allow further documentation to occur in any record involved in litigation

83. The Breach Notification Rule requires covered entities to establish a process for investigating whether a breach has occurred and which of the following?

a. Establish a new position for a Privacy Officer

b. Notify affected individuals when a breach occurs

c. Establish a policy on minimum necessary

d. Notify the primary care physicians of all patients of the breach

84. The HIPAA methods titled Expert Determination and Safe Harbor are ways in which the following can be achieved legally.

a. Data analysis

b. Reidentification

c. Deidentification

d. Public health reporting

85. Placing locks on computer room doors is considered what type of security control?

a. Electronic access control

b. Workstation control

c. Physical access control

d. Security breach

86. Anywhere General Hospital allows all of the ICU nurses to log on with a standard ID and password. This is not allowed by which standard of the Security Rule?

a. Workforce Security Standard

b. Workstation Security Standard

c. Authorization Control Standard

d. Access Control Standard

Domain 3 *Informatics, Analytics, and Data Use*

87. A request for proposal (RFP) serves two important purposes: it solidifies the planning information and healthcare entity requirements into a single document, and it:

 a. Allows one vendor an advantage over the other potential vendors
 b. Delineates the entity's system requirements in such a way that a vendor is selected without review of the entire RFP pool
 c. Enables the healthcare entity to make decisions quickly
 d. Provides valuable insights into the vendors operations and products and levels the playing field in terms of asking all the vendors the same questions

88. A possible justification for building an information system in-house rather than purchasing one from a vendor is that:

 a. It is cheaper to buy than to build
 b. The facility has development teams they do not want to give up
 c. Integration of systems will be easier
 d. Vendor products are not comprehensive enough

89. What is the formatting problem in the following table?

Medical Center Hospital Admission Types		
Elective	2,843	62.4
Emergency admission	942	37.6
Total	3,785	100.0

 a. The variable names are missing
 b. The title of the table is missing
 c. The column headings are missing
 d. The column totals are inaccurate

90. Community Memorial Hospital had 25 inpatient deaths, including newborns, during the month of June. The hospital had a total of 500 discharges for the same period, including deaths of adults, children, and newborns. The hospital's gross death rate for the month of June was:

 a. 0.05%
 b. 2%
 c. 5%
 d. 20%

91. In which of the following phases of systems selection and implementation would the process of running a mock query to assess the functionality of a database be performed?

 a. Initial study
 b. Design
 c. Testing
 d. Operation

92. You want to graph the average length of stay by sex and service for the month of April. Which graphic tool would you use?

a. Bar graph

b. Histogram

c. Line graph

d. Pie chart

93. In healthcare, a data warehouse may be use for:

a. Accounts receivable management

b. Materials or inventory management

c. Best practice guideline development

d. Utilization review

94. If an analyst is studying the wait times at a clinic and the only list of patients available is on hard copy, which sampling technique is the easiest to use?

a. Survey sampling

b. Systematic sampling

c. Cluster sampling

d. Stratified sampling

95. To reduce the effect of a server crash in an EHR environment, it is advisable to:

a. Set up redundant systems

b. Have a storage area network

c. Store data in RAID

d. Have an inventory of all systems

96. In assessing the quality of care given to patients with diabetes mellitus, the quality team collects data regarding blood sugar levels on admission and on discharge. This data is called a(n):

a. Indicator

b. Measurement

c. Assessment

d. Outcome

97. By querying the healthcare entity data, you find that patients admitted on a weekend have a mean length of stay that is 1.3 days longer than patients who are admitted Monday through Friday. This method of finding information is called:

a. Structuring query language

b. Data mining

c. Multidimensional data structuring

d. Satisficing

98. A health information professional is preparing statistical information about the third-party payers that reimburse care in the facility. She finds the following information: Medicare reimburses 46 percent; Medicaid reimburses 13 percent; Blue Cross reimburses 21 percent; workers' compensation reimburses 1 percent; commercial plans reimburse 15 percent; and other payers or self-payers reimburse 4 percent. What is the best graphic tool to use to display this data?

a. Histogram

b. Pie chart

c. Line graph

d. Table

99. During an influenza outbreak, a nursing home reports 25 new cases of influenza in a given month. These 25 cases represent 30 percent of the nursing home's population. This rate represents the:

a. Distribution

b. Frequency

c. Incidence

d. Prevalence

100. The researcher's informed consent form stated that the patients' information would be anonymous. Later, in the application form for Institutional Review Board (IRB) approval, the researcher described a coding system to track respondents and nonrespondents. The IRB returned the application to the researcher with the stipulation that the informed consent must be changed. What raised the red flag?

a. The description of the use of a coding system to track respondents and nonrespondents

b. The application form for the IRB approval

c. The researcher's informed consent form

d. The description of the use of a coding system to track respondents

101. The following data have been collected by the hospital quality council. What conclusions can be made from the data on the hospital's quality of care between the first and second quarters?

Measure	1st Qtr	2nd Qtr
Medication errors	3.2%	10.4%
Patient falls	4.2%	8.6%
Hospital-acquired infections	1.8%	4.9%
Transfusion reactions	1.4%	2.5%

a. Quality of care improved between the first and second quarters.

b. Quality of care is about the same between the first and second quarters.

c. Quality of care is declining between the first and second quarters.

d. Quality of care should not be judged by these types of measures.

102. Using the admission criteria provided, determine if the following patient meets the severity of illness and intensity of service criteria for admission.

Severity of Illness	Intensity of Service
Persistent fever	Inpatient-approved surgery/procedure within 24 hours of admission
Active bleeding	Intravenous medications or fluid replacement
Wound dehiscence	Vital signs every 2 hours or more often

Sue presents with vaginal bleeding. An ultrasound showed a missed abortion so she is being admitted to the outpatient surgery suite for a D&C.

a. The patient does not meet both severity of illness and intensity of service criteria.
b. The patient does meet both severity of illness and intensity of service criteria.
c. The patient meets intensity of service criteria but not severity of illness.
d. The patient meets severity of illness criteria but not intensity of service.

103. Which of the following is ***not*** true of a PHR?

a. Individuals own and manage their PHR
b. It is a life-long resource
c. Individuals determine rights of access
d. It will replace the legal records of providers

104. For the following excerpt from a patient satisfaction survey, determine if in the development of this survey the designer is adhering to good survey design principles.

What is your zip code? _______		
Sex (circle one):	Male	Female
What is your age?		
0–17 _______	_______	_______
18–35 _______	_______	_______
36–45 _______	_______	_______
46–60 _______	_______	_______

a. All survey design principles were applied in the development of this survey.
b. The survey design principle of consistent format was applied in the development of this survey.
c. The survey design principle of mutually exclusive categories was applied in the development of this survey.
d. The survey design principles were not applied in the development of this survey.

105. In carrying out the strategic plan for health IT, the step that describes what is needed to achieve the plan's goals is:

a. Environmental scan
b. Project plan
c. Requirements analysis
d. Risk analysis

106. Community Memorial Hospital discharged nine patients on April 1. The length of stay for each patient is shown in the following table. The average length of stay for these nine patients was:

Patient	Number of Days
A	1
B	5
C	3
D	3
E	8
F	8
G	8
H	9
I	9

a. 5 days

b. 6 days

c. 8 days

d. 9 days

107. What type of data display tool is used to display discrete categories?

a. Bar graph

b. Histogram

c. Pie chart

d. Line chart

108. Assume you are the manager of a 10-physician group primary care practice. The physicians are interested in contracting with an application service provider to develop and manage patient records electronically. Which of the following statements is an indication that an application service provider (ASP) may be a good idea for this practice?

a. The practice does not have the up-front capital or IT staff needed to purchase and implement a system from a health information systems vendor.

b. The practice wants an electronic medical record system and wants to get into the IT management business as well.

c. The practice would like to have the system up and running in a relatively short period of time (less than four months).

d. The practice is not looking to purchase any additional hardware needed for an electronic medical record system.

109. The application of information science to the management of healthcare data and information through computer technology is referred to as:

a. Data definitions

b. Data resource management

c. Healthcare informatics

d. Clinical information systems

110. This Health Information Exchange (HIE) consent model requires the patient to give their consent for the inclusion of their data in the HIE.

a. Opt-in

b. Opt-out

c. Automatic consent

d. No-consent

111. The use of electronic information and telecommunications technologies to support long-distance clinical healthcare, patient and professional health-related education, public health, and health administration is called:

a. Secure messaging

b. Consumer informatics

c. Personalized medicine

d. Telehealth

112. Given the information here, the case-mix index would be:

MS-DRG	MDC	Type	MS-DRG Title	Weight	Discharges	Geometric Mean	Arithmetic Mean
191	04	MED	Chronic obstructive pulmonary disease w CC	0.9321	10	3.3	4.0
192	04	MED	Chronic obstructive pulmonary disease w/o CC/MCC	0.7313	20	22.7	3.3
193	04	MED	Simple pneumonia & pleurisy w MCC	1.4261	10	44.8	55.8
194	04	MED	Simple pneumonia & pleurisy w CC	0.9695	20	3.7	4.4
195	04	MED	Simple pneumonia & pleurisy w/o CC/MCC	0.7111	10	2.8	3.3

a. 0.07

b. 0.644

c. 0.9244

d. 64.7

113. Which of the following activities is likely to occur in the analysis phase of the systems development life cycle?

a. Examine the current system and identify opportunities for improvement

b. Send out RFPs to prospective vendors

c. Negotiate a contract with the vendor

d. Install necessary hardware and software

114. At Medical Center Hospital, the master patient index system is not meeting facility needs. There are duplicate numbers and errors in patient identification information. The IS director replaces the system with a newer system from a different vendor. After several months, the new system is exhibiting many of the same problems as the old system, and the facility staff is frustrated and angry. What is the most likely cause of the problem?

a. The new system has the same design flaws as the previous system.

b. The old system was not properly disabled and has infected the new system.

c. Underlying human and process problems were not identified and corrected prior to making a system change.

d. Human error is the cause of all of the problems with both systems.

115. Which of the following do HIE participants use to search for health records on other healthcare organization systems using patient indexing and identification software?

a. Admit, discharge, transfer

b. Advance patient identifier

c. Continuity of care document

d. Record locator service

116. Which of the following would likely be recorded on an information systems issues log?

a. Alan is present every day there is a system test.

b. Betty reported receiving 25 erroneous e-mail messages.

c. Dr. Brown effectively uses e-prescribing.

d. John requested a supply of tamperproof paper for his office.

117. How are Hospital Compare measures used by CMS?

a. Hospitals that score better than average receive bonus payments.

b. Hospitals that report all measures receive the full payment update.

c. Hospitals that perform poorly must pay a penalty.

d. Hospital payment is not impacted by hospital compare indicators.

118. John Smith, who was treated as a patient at a multihospital system, has three medical record numbers. The term used to describe multiple health record numbers is:

a. Duplicates

b. Overlay

c. Overlap

d. Integrity

119. HIM departments may be the hub of identifying, mitigating, and correcting master patient index (MPI) errors. But that information often is not shared with other departments within the healthcare entity. After identifying procedural problems that contribute to the creation of the MPI errors, which department should the MPI manager work with to correct these procedural problems?

a. Administration

b. Registration or patient access

c. Risk management

d. Radiology and laboratory

120. Technology that electronically stores, manages, and distributes documents that are generated in a digital format and whose output data are report-formatted and print-stream originated is called:

a. Business process management (BPM) technology

b. Automated forms processing technology

c. Computer output laser disk (COLD) technology

d. Digital signature management technology

121. University Medical Center contracts with the XYZ Corporation for a clinical information system. The hospital pays a fixed monthly fee. XYZ owns the hardware and hosts the application software using the Internet. The Medical Center accesses the system through onsite workstations. In this situation, XYZ Corporation is a(n):

a. Application service provider

b. Neural network

c. Health information system database

d. Clinician portal

122. What kind of data might be displayed on a pie chart?

a. Average length of stay by year

b. Percentage of discharges by third-party payer

c. Number of discharges per year by third-party payer

d. Number of patients discharged by sex and service

123. What type of authentication is created when a person signs his or her name on a pen pad and the signature is automatically converted and affixed to a computer document?

a. Digital signature

b. Electronic validation

c. Electronic signature

d. Digital authorization key

124. Using the staff turnover information in this graph, determine the next action the quality council at this hospital should take.

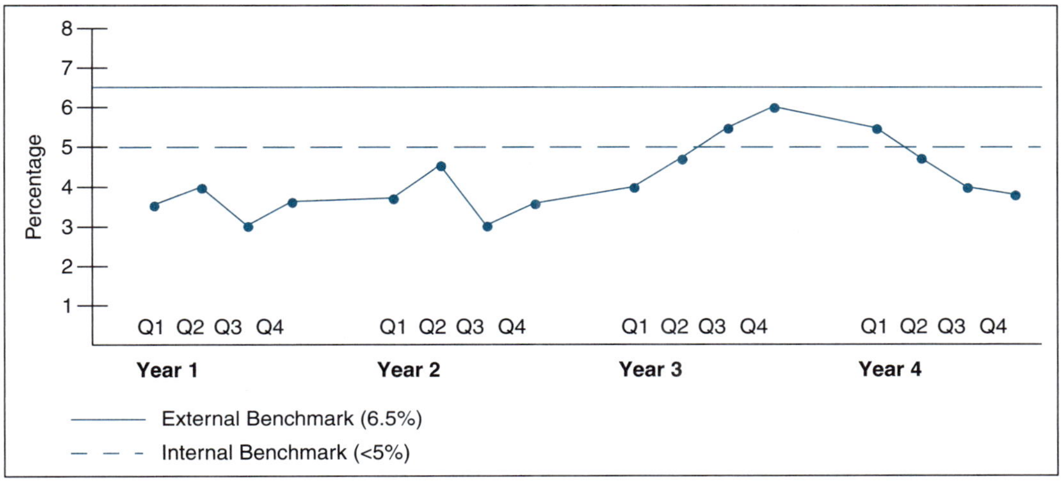

a. Do nothing, as the data is below the external benchmark

b. Coordinate a PI team to look into the cause for the high employee turnover rate in year 3

c. Coordinate a PI team to look into the cause for the drop in employee turnover rate in year 4

d. Do nothing, as the data is above the internal benchmark

125. The Joint Commission and CMS identify core measures that provide an indication of a healthcare facility's performance. Some of the core measure data sets include which of the following?

a. Myocardial infarction, pneumonia, and HIV/AIDS

b. Pneumonia, congestive heart failure, and gastric ulcers

c. Pneumonia, congestive heart failure, and myocardial infarction

d. Congestive heart failure, HIV/AIDS, and myocardial infarction

126. The MPI manager has identified a pattern of duplicate health record numbers from the specimen processing area of the hospital. After spending time merging the patient information and correcting the duplicates in the patient information system, the MPI manager needs to notify which department to correct the source system data?

a. Laboratory

b. Radiology

c. Quality management

d. Registration

127. It is impossible to have health information interoperability or health information exchange without the following:

a. 100 percent adoption of EHRs

b. A federally mandated Data Use and Reciprocal Support Agreement

c. Complete, publicly available standards

d. ONC and CMS regulations

128. The technology commonly utilized for automated claims processing (sending bills directly to third-party payers) is:

a. Optical character recognition
b. Bar coding
c. Neural networks
d. Electronic data interchange

129. If an analyst wishes to predict future ancillary charges for hip replacement patients based on the age of the patient, which of the following is a correct statement?

a. Age is the dependent variable; ancillary charges is the independent variable.
b. Age is the independent variable; ancillary charges is the dependent variable.
c. The average ancillary charge is the best estimator,
d. The two variables cannot be related.

Domain 4 *Revenue Management*

130. Medical identity thefts are situations in which the following occurs:

a. When health information on the wrong patient is put in the incorrect record
b. When financial information is used to purchase nonmedical items
c. When demographic and financial information is used to acquire medical services
d. When demographic information is used to purchase nonmedical items

131. The practice of using a code that results in a higher payment to the provider than the code that actually reflects the service or item provided is known as:

a. Unbundling
b. Billing for services not provided
c. Medically unnecessary services
d. Upcoding

132. You are the coding supervisor and you are doing an audit of outpatient coding. Robert Thompson was seen in the outpatient department with a chronic cough and the record states, "rule out lung cancer." What should have been coded as the patient's diagnosis?

a. Chronic cough
b. Observation and evaluation without need for further medical care
c. Diagnosis of unknown etiology
d. Lung cancer

133. Using the following custom revenue production report, which coding error may be demonstrated in the report?

Revenue Production Report—Small Multispecialty Group Month: January				
Code	Quantity	Fee	Projected Revenue	Actual Insurance Revenue
99201	0	$50	$0	$0.00
99202	3	$75	$225	$164.10
99203	4	$90	$360	$267.94
99204	0	$120	$0	$0.00
99205	0	$150	$0	$0.00
99211	703	$28	$19,684	$14,988.32
99212	489	$47	$22,983	$18,092.65
99213	1853	$63	$116,739	$92,890.38
99214	41	$89	$3,649	$2,799.11
99215	7	$135	$945	$722.87
99241	3	$100	$300	$52.50
99242	9	$125	$1,125	$156.23
99243	27	$150	$4,050	$610.45
99244	10	$175	$1,750	$124.32
99245	1	$200	$200	$53.10

a. Clustering
b. Unbundling
c. Missed charges
d. Overcoding

134. Before Central Hospital is permitted to open and provide medical services in a particular state, the healthcare entity must first go through which of the following processes?

a. Accreditation
b. Licensure
c. Qualification
d. Certification

135. The health plan reimburses Dr. Tan $15 per patient per month. In January, Dr. Tan saw 300 patients so he received $4,500 from the health plan. What method is the health plan using to reimburse Dr. Tan?

a. Traditional retrospective
b. Capitated rate
c. Relative value
d. Discounted fee schedule

136. For Medicare patients, how often must the home health agency's assessment and care plan be updated?

a. At least every 60 days or as often as the severity of the patient's condition requires

b. Every 30 days

c. As often as the severity of the patient's condition requires

d. Every 60 days

137. A physician performed a total abdominal hysterectomy with bilateral salpingo-oophorectomy on his patient at Community Hospital. His office billed the following:

58150	Total abdominal hysterectomy (corpus and cervix), with or without removal of tube(s), with or without removal of ovary(s)
58720	Salpingo-oophorectomy, complete or partial, unilateral or bilateral (separate procedure)

Why was this claim rejected?

a. Billed hysterectomy with wrong CPT code

b. Not a covered procedure

c. Unbundled procedures

d. Covered procedure but insurance company requires additional information

138. A patient saw a neurosurgeon for treatment of a nerve that was severed in an industrial accident. The patient worked for Basic Manufacturing Company where the industrial accident occurred. Basic Manufacturing carried workers' compensation insurance. The workers' compensation insurance paid the neurosurgeon fees. Which entity is the "third party"?

a. Patient

b. Neurosurgeon

c. Basic Manufacturing Company

d. Workers' compensation insurance

139. A physician query may not be appropriate in which of the following instances?

a. Diagnosis of viral pneumonia noted in the progress notes and sputum cultures showing *Haemophilus influenzae*

b. Discharge summary indicates chronic renal failure but the progress notes document acute renal failure throughout the stay

c. Acute respiratory failure in a patient whose lab report findings appear to not support this diagnosis

d. Diagnosis of chest pain and abnormal cardiac enzymes indicative of an AMI

140. The financial manager of the physician group practice explained that the healthcare insurance company would be reimbursing the practice for its treatment of the exacerbation of congestive heart failure that Mrs. Zale experienced. The exacerbation, treatment, and resolution covered approximately five weeks. The payment covered all the services that Mrs. Zale incurred during the period. What method of reimbursement was the physician group practice receiving?

a. Traditional

b. Episode-of-care

c. Per diem

d. Fee-for-service

141. The practice of undercoding can affect a hospital's MS-DRG case mix in which of the following ways?

a. Makes it lower than warranted by the actual service or resource intensity of the facility
b. Makes it higher than warranted by the actual service or resource intensity of the facility
c. Does not affect the hospital's MS-DRG case mix
d. Coding has nothing to do with a hospital's MS-DRG case mix

142. The following table is an example of an:

Patient/ Service	Service Date(s)	(A) Total Charge	(B) Not Payable by Plan		Plan Paid Amount	
White, Jane						
Office Visit	02/17/201X	$56.00	$10.00	CP*	$46.00	100%
X-Ray	02/17/201X	$268.00	$250.00 $3.60	DD* CI*	$14.40	80%
Lab	02/17/201X	$20.00	$15.00	CP*	$5.00	100%
Total						

**CI: Coinsurance; CP: Copayment; DD: Deductible*

a. Insurance coverage advanced notice service waiver
b. Explanation of benefits
c. Insurance claim form
d. Encounter form

143. Which of the following healthcare entities' mission is to reduce Medicare improper payments through detection and collection of overpayments, identification of underpayments, and implementation of actions that will prevent future improper payments?

a. Accountable care entity
b. Managed care entity
c. Revenue reduction contractor
d. Recovery audit contractor

144. Which of the following conditions would be the most likely to fall into the category of notifiable diseases as defined by the National Notifiable Diseases Surveillance System?

a. Diabetes mellitus
b. Coronary artery disease
c. Fracture of major bones
d. HIV infection

145. The coding manager at Community Hospital is seeing an increased number of physicians failing to document the cause and effect of diabetes and its manifestations. Which of the following will provide the most comprehensive solution to handle this documentation issue?

a. Have coders continue to query the attending physician for this documentation.
b. Present this information at the next medical staff meeting to inform physicians on documentation standards and guidelines.
c. Do nothing because coding compliance guidelines do not allow any action.
d. Place all offending physicians on suspension if the documentation issues continue.

146. A coder notes that the patient is taking prescribed Haldol. The final diagnoses on the progress notes include diabetes mellitus, acute pharyngitis, and malnutrition. What condition might the coder suspect the patient has that the physician should be queried to confirm?

a. Insomnia
b. Hypertension
c. Mental or behavior problems
d. Rheumatoid arthritis

147. In conducting a qualitative review, the clinical documentation specialist sees that the nursing staff has documented the patient's skin integrity on admission to support the presence of a stage I pressure ulcer. However, the physician's documentation is unclear as to whether this condition was present on admission. How should the clinical documentation specialist proceed?

a. Note the condition as present on admission
b. Query the physician to determine if the condition was present on admission
c. Note the condition as unknown on admission
d. Note the condition as not present on admission

148. Phil White had coronary artery bypass graft surgery. Unfortunately, during the surgery, Phil suffered a severe stroke. Phil's recovery included several settings in the continuum of care: acute-care hospital, physician office, rehabilitation center, and home health agency. This initial service and subsequent recovery lasted 10 months. As a member of a managed care organization in an integrated delivery system, how should Phil expect that his healthcare billing will be handled?

a. Bills for each service from each physician, each facility, and each other healthcare provider from every encounter
b. Bills for each service from each physician, each facility, and each other healthcare provider at the end of the 10-month period
c. Consolidated billing for each encounter that includes the bills from all the physicians, facilities, and other healthcare providers involved in the encounter
d. One fixed amount for the entire episode that is divided among all the physicians, facilities, and other healthcare providers

149. The coding supervisor has compiled a report on the number of coding errors made each day by the coding staff. The report data show that Tim makes an average of six errors per day, Jane makes an average of five errors per day, and Bob and Susan each make an average of two errors per day. Given this information, what action should the coding supervisor take?

a. Counsel Tim and Jane because they have the highest error rates
b. Encourage Tim and Jane to get additional training
c. Provide Bob and Susan with incentive pay for low coding error rates
d. Take no action since not enough information is given to make a judgment

150. Once all data has been posted to patient's account, the claim can be reviewed for accuracy and completeness. Many facilities have an internal auditing system that runs each claim through a set of edits. This internal auditing system is known as a:

a. Chargemaster
b. Superbill
c. Scrubber
d. Grouper

151. Which of the following payment arrangements is streamlined by the use of chargemasters?

a. Fee-for-service
b. Per diem
c. Prospective
d. Retrospective

152. Which of the following would generally be found in a query to a physician?

a. Health record number and demographic information
b. Name and contact number of the individual initiating the query and account number
c. Date query initiated and date query must be completed
d. Demographic information and name and contact number of individual initiating the query

153. A ________ assists in educating medical staff members on documentation needed for accurate billing.

a. Physician advisor
b. Compliance officer
c. Chargemaster coordinator
d. Data monitor

Domain 5 *Leadership*

154. A director of health information services in a hospital wants to implement a computer-based patient record system over the next 2 years. She gets support from the CIO, who advocates for the project with the administrative team. The CIO has become the project's _____.

a. Stakeholder
b. Champion
c. Manager
d. Owner

155. External change agents have the advantage over internal agents regarding:

a. Benchmarking the healthcare entity against other entities
b. Being less objective
c. Understanding the history of the entity
d. Being less expensive to employ

156. The slightly higher wage paid to an employee who works a less desirable shift is called a:

a. Shift rotation
b. Performance incentive
c. Shift differential
d. Work distribution ladder

157. According to the records kept on filing unit performance over the past year, the filing unit has filed an average of 1,000 records per day. You have three full-time equivalent (FTE) record filers in the department who are productive 88 percent of each workday (that is, 12 percent unproductive or 12 percent PFD). Based on this information, what is the average number of records filed per productive hour in the file unit as a whole?

a. 42 records per hour

b. 48 records per hour

c. 110 records per hour

d. 143 records per hour

158. Reviewing the following PERT chart, what is the critical path for this project?

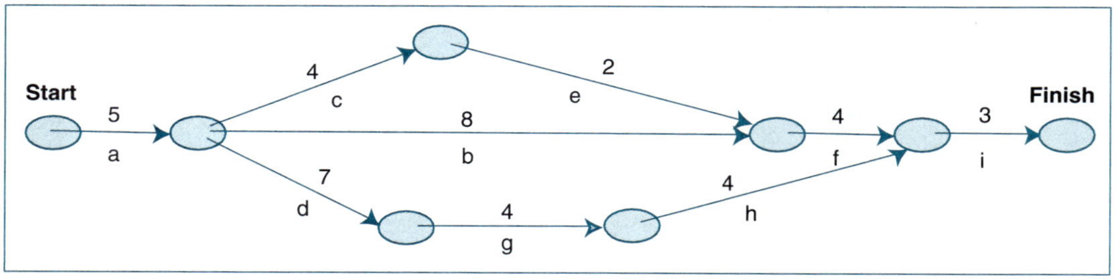

a. a → c → d → f → i

b. a → b → f → i

c. a → d → g → h → i

d. a → c → e → f → i

159. Employees covered by the provisions of the Fair Labor Standards Act (FLSA) are called ________ employees.

a. Waged

b. Salaried

c. Exempt

d. Nonexempt

160. A technique for measuring healthcare entity performance across the four perspectives of customer, financial, internal processes, and learning and growth is called:

a. Strategy map

b. Process innovations

c. Balanced scorecard methodology

d. SWOT analysis

161. The financial statement that presents a record of operations by showing revenue and expenses over a period of time is called the:

a. Balance sheet

b. Statement of cash flows

c. Income statement

d. Statement of retained earnings

162. The HIM department records copy fees as revenue. For the year the budgeted fees were $25,000 and the actual fees received are $23,000. The director may be asked to explain a(n):

a. Favorable variance of $2,000

b. Unfavorable variance of $2,000

c. Favorable variance of $23,000

d. Unfavorable variance of $23,000

163. Joe Smith, RHIA, works for an outsourcing company as interim health information department director in a large hospital. By the terms of the contract, the hospital pays the company for Joe's services based on a 40-hour workweek with overtime for any hours exceeding 40. Joe typically works 9 hours per day, Monday through Thursday, and 4 hours on Friday. He then flies home for the weekend. After several months, he discovers the hospital is billed for 44 to 48 hours per week almost every week. Joe confronts the company billing department because this practice conflicts with the tenet of the AHIMA Code of Ethics that states that health information management professionals:

a. Respect the rights and dignity of all individuals

b. Adhere to the vision, mission, and values of the association

c. Promote and protect the confidentiality and security of health records and health information

d. Refuse to participate in or conceal unethical practices or procedures

164. Which of the following statements is most accurate regarding effective communication?

a. Use passive listening

b. Monitor others' nonverbal behaviors for cues that they are following or confused

c. Make sure all parties are distracted to better communicate your message

d. Message content is more important than how it is delivered

165. Which of the following would be an indicator of process problems in a health information department?

a. 5% decline in the number of patients who indicate satisfaction with hospital care

b. 10% increase in the average length of stay

c. 15% reduction in bed turnover rate

d. 18% error rate on abstracting data

166. Which of the following is a true statement about business process reengineering?

a. It is intended to make small incremental changes to improve a process.

b. It seeks to reevaluate and redesign organizational processes to make dramatic performance improvements.

c. It implies making few changes to achieve significant improvements in cost, quality, service, and speed.

d. Its main focus is to reduce services.

167. Strategic thinkers exhibit which of the following skills?

a. Discomfort with uncertainty and risk

b. The ability to gain a powerful core of healthcare entity supporters and customers

c. Flexibility but lacking creativity

d. An ability to implement the vision and plan and be uncomfortable with change

168. The form of coaching in which an individual in the beginning stages of a career is matched with a senior person is known as:

a. Cross-training
b. Mentoring
c. Orientation
d. Motivation

169. A set of activities designed to familiarize new employees with their jobs, the healthcare entity, and work culture is called:

a. Training
b. Job analysis
c. Orientation
d. Job rotation

170. Which of the following statements is most accurate regarding the relationship between levels of management and managerial skills?

a. Interpersonal skills increase as one goes from lower to upper management
b. Technological skills are greatest at the top level of management
c. Conceptual skills are greatest at the top level of management
d. Interpersonal, technical, and conceptual skills are required in equal amounts at all levels of the healthcare entity

171. A director of health information services in a hospital wants to implement a computer-based patient record system over the next two years. She gets support from the CIO, who champions the project with the administrative team. The CIO has become the project's:

a. Stakeholder
b. Sponsor
c. Manager
d. Budget director

172. The following information was abstracted from Community Hospital's balance sheet.

Total assets	$25,000,000
Current assets	$4,000,000
Total liabilities	$10,000,000
Current liabilities	$5,000,000

A vendor selling a large dollar amount of goods to this hospital on credit would:

a. Not be concerned because total assets exceed total liabilities
b. Not be concerned because the debt ratio is less than one half
c. Be somewhat concerned because the current ratio is less than one
d. Not analyze the balance sheet because the vendor would care more about the income statement

173. Community Hospital is evaluating the following three investments. Which one has the highest profitability index?

	Radiology Investment	Cardiology Investment	Pharmacy Investment
Present value of cash inflows	$2,000,000	$1,200,000	$40,000
Present value of cash outflows	$500,000	$300,000	$10,000

a. Radiology investment

b. Cardiology investment

c. Pharmacy investment

d. All three are equally profitable

174. The advantage of using internal change agents over external change agents is that the former can usually:

a. Be accepted by employees as being more objective

b. More easily challenge healthcare entity norms and culture

c. Benchmark the healthcare entity against others

d. Provide a more detailed understanding of healthcare entity's history and issues

175. The performance standard to "respond to release of information requests for continuing care in one working day 95 percent of the time" is an example of a:

a. Qualitative standard

b. Quantitative standard

c. Joint Commission standard

d. Compliance standard

176. In the following figure, identify the component of the project plan labeled as B.

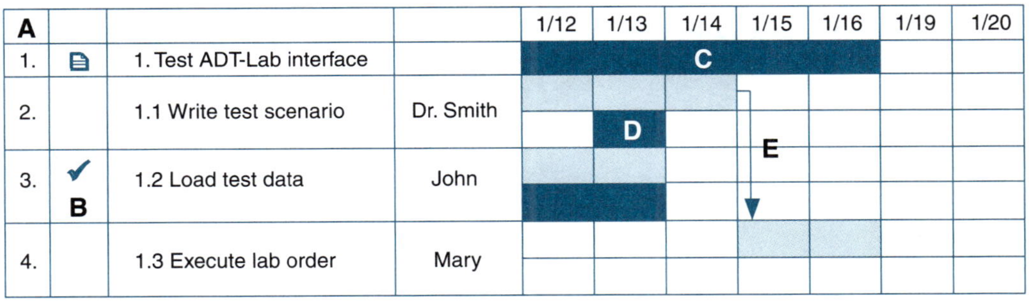

a. Row numbers

b. Task completed

c. Task progress

d. Dependency

177. Which of the following is the best reason for team building?

a. To quickly move from acquaintanceship to a strong team

b. To identify a leader

c. To help employees develop a common purpose

d. To ensure that the leader's situation is favorable

178. Contracting for staffing to handle a complete function within the HIM department, such as the Cancer Registry function, would be considered what type of contracting arrangement?

a. Full-service

b. Part-time

c. Project-based

d. Temporary

179. Every year, a director of health information services sponsors a series of presentations about the confidentiality of patient information. All facility employees are required to attend a session. This method of educational delivery is called:

a. Career development

b. In-service education

c. On-the-job training

d. Orientation

180. A transcription manager is assigned to a project team that is implementing a voice recognition system. He reports to the director of health information services for regular job functions and to the project manager for tasks related to the project. This is an example of which type of project management structure?

a. Strong matrixed

b. Projectized

c. Functional

d. Weak matrixed

PRACTICE EXAM 2

Domain 1 *Data Content, Structure, and Standards*

1. Mary Smith, RHIA, has been asked to work on the development of a hospital trauma data registry. Which of the following data sets would be most helpful in developing this registry?

   a. DEEDS

   b. MDS

   c. OASIS

   d. UACDS

2. Who owns the health records of patients treated in a healthcare facility?

   a. The patient

   b. The third-party payer

   c. The facility

   d. The patient's family

3. In figuring a drug dosage, it is unacceptable to round up to the nearest gram if the drug is to be dosed in milligrams. Which dimension of data quality is being applied in this situation?

   a. Accuracy

   b. Granularity

   c. Precision

   d. Currency

4. Legally, which of the following is most important in determining the length of time a hospital must retain health records?

   a. Research needs

   b. Storage capabilities

   c. Statute of limitations

   d. Cost

5. The health information management (HIM) manager is concerned with a backlog in transcription of surgical reports. The medical staff rules and regulations stipulate that the surgeon should:

   a. Wait for the transcribed report

   b. Re-dictate the operative report

   c. Write a detailed postoperative progress note about the procedure performed

   d. Write a postoperative progress note that states the operative report has been dictated

6. One member of the medical staff reviewed a patient's history, examined the patient, and wrote findings and recommendations at the request of another member of the medical staff. The resulting medical report that documents the response of the reviewing medical staff member is a:

   a. Consultation report

   b. Discharge report

   c. History and physical exam

   d. Pathology report

7. The discharge summary must be completed within ________ after discharge for most patients but within ________ for patients transferred to other facilities. Discharge summaries are not always required for patients who were hospitalized for less than ________ hours.

   a. 30 days, 48 hours, 24 hours
   b. 14 days, 24 hours, 48 hours
   c. 14 days, 48 hours, 24 hours
   d. 30 days, 24 hours, 48 hours

8. Burning, shredding, pulping, and pulverizing are all acceptable methods in which process?

   a. Deidentification of electronic documents
   b. Destruction of paper-based health records
   c. Deidentification of records stored on microfilm
   d. Destruction of computer-based health records

9. Which of the following would be the best approach in starting a data governance program?

   a. Focus on one or a few small business imperatives
   b. Begin with developing policies and procedures
   c. Identify HIPAA requirements
   d. Establish success metrics

10. A health record that maintains information throughout the lifespan of the patient, ideally from birth to death, is known as a:

   a. Problem-oriented health record
   b. Patient-centric record
   c. Longitudinal health record
   d. Health record

11. Who is responsible for the content, quality, and signing of the discharge summary?

   a. Attending physician
   b. Head nurse
   c. Consulting physician
   d. Admitting nurse

12. Under which circumstances may an interval note be added to a patient's health record in place of a complete history and physical?

   a. When the patient is readmitted a second time for the same condition
   b. When the patient is readmitted within 30 days of the initial treatment for a different condition
   c. When the patient is readmitted a third time for the same condition
   d. When the patient is readmitted within 30 days of the initial treatment for the same condition

13. The procedure that was performed for the definitive treatment (rather than the diagnosis) of the main condition or a complication of the condition is the:

   a. Chief procedure
   b. Principal treatment
   c. Comorbidity
   d. Principal procedure

14. An HIM professional who is designing a health record system for a healthcare entity should check ________ to find out how long health records should be retained by the entity.

a. with the attending physician

b. state and federal law

c. county or city codes

d. Joint Commission Accreditation Standards

15. The clinical statement "microscopic sections of the gallbladder reveal a surface lined by tall columnar cells of uniform size and shape" would be documented on which health record form?

a. Operative report

b. Pathology report

c. Discharge summary

d. Nursing note

16. Standardizing medical terminology to avoid differences in naming various medical conditions and procedures (such as the synonyms bunionectomy, McBride procedure, and repair of hallux valgus) is one purpose of:

a. Content and structure standards

b. Security standards

c. Transaction standards

d. Vocabulary standards

17. As part of the initiative to improve data integrity, the Data Quality Committee conducted an inventory of all the hospital's databases. The review showed that more than 70 percent of the identified databases did not have data dictionaries. Given this data, what should be the committee's first action?

a. Disregard the data

b. Establish a data dictionary policy with associated standards

c. Develop an in-service training program on data dictionary use

d. Distribute a memorandum to all department heads on the value of a data dictionary

18. What relationships is the following entity relationship diagram showing?

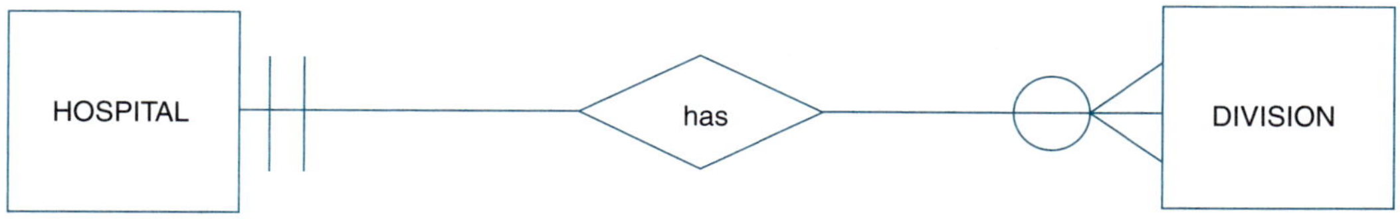

a. Each division has one hospital, but each hospital has many divisions.

b. Each hospital has one division, but each division has many hospitals.

c. Each hospital has one division, and each division has one hospital.

d. Each division has one hospital, and each hospital has one division.

19. To meet meaningful use standards, Anywhere Hospital is implementing a document imaging system and electronic document management system. This is an interim step before full implementation of computerized provider order entry and point-of-care documentation. This step-by-step process is part of Anywhere Hospital's:

a. Migration plan

b. Strategic plan

c. Bylaws update

d. Regulatory update

20. Assign codes for the following scenario: A 35-year-old male is admitted with esophageal reflux. An esophagoscopy and closed esophageal biopsy was performed.

K20.9	Esophagitis, unspecified
K21.0	Gastro-esophageal reflux disease with esophagitis
K21.9	Gastro-esophageal reflux disease without esophagitis

Section	Body System	Root Operation	Body Part	Approach	Device	Qualifier
Medical and Surgical	Gastrointestinal System	Inspection	Upper Intestinal Tract	Via Natural or Artificial Opening Endoscopic	No Device	No Qualifier
0	D	J	0	8	Z	Z

Section	Body System	Root Operation	Body Part	Approach	Device	Qualifier
Medical and Surgical	Gastrointestinal System	Excision	Esophagus	Via Natural or Artificial Opening Endoscopic	No Device	Diagnostic
0	D	B	5	8	Z	X

Section	Body System	Root Operation	Body Part	Approach	Device	Qualifier
Medical and Surgical	Gastrointestinal System	Excision	Esophagus	Via Natural or Artificial Opening Endoscopic	No Device	No Qualifier
0	D	B	5	8	Z	Z

a. K21.9, 0DB58ZX

b. K20.9, 0DB58ZZ

c. K21.0, 0DB58ZX

d. K21.9, 0DJ08ZZ, 0DB58ZX

21. Which of the following statements does not pertain to paper-based health records?

   a. They are kept in locked storage areas that are accessible only to authorized staff.
   b. They are logged out according to the healthcare entity's prescribed procedure.
   c. They are forwarded to the appropriate service area when needed for patient care purposes.
   d. They have a built-in access control mechanism.

22. A number assigned to patients in a cancer registry in the order that the patients are entered in the registry every year (for example, 03-0001) is a(n) ________ number.

   a. Accession
   b. Reference
   c. Follow-up
   d. Tracking

23. Which method of documenting physician progress notes is ***not*** acceptable for meeting documentation standards?

   a. Narrative note
   b. Flowchart
   c. Computer input
   d. Charting by exception

24. Using the information in these partial attribute lists for the PATIENT, VISIT, and CLINIC columns in a relational database, the attribute PATIENT_MRN is listed in both the PATIENT Entity Attributes and the VISIT Entity Attributes, and CLINIC_ID is listed in both the VISIT Entity Attributes and the CLINIC Entity Attributes. What does the attribute CLINIC_ID represent?

PATIENT Entity Attributes

PATIENT_MRN (PK)
PATIENT_LNAME
PATIENT_FNAME
PATIENT_MNAME
PATIENT_STREET
PATIENT_CITY
PATIENT_STATE
PATIENT_ZIPCODE
PATIENT_PHONE
PATIENT_DOB
. . .

VISIT Entity Attributes

VISIT_ID (PK)
VISIT_DATE
VISIT_REASON
PATIENT_MRN (FK)
CLINIC_ID (FK)
. . .

CLINIC Entity Attributes

CLINIC_ID (PK)
CLINIC_NAME
CLINIC_STREET
CLINIC_CITY
CLINIC_STATE
CLINIC_ZIPCODE
CLINIC_PHONE
CLINIC_FAX
. . .

   a. It is the foreign key in CLINIC and the primary key in VISIT.
   b. It is the primary key in CLINIC and the foreign key in VISIT.
   c. It is the primary key in both CLINIC and VISIT.
   d. It is the foreign key in both CLINIC and VISIT.

25. Two clerks are abstracting data for a registry. When their work is checked, discrepancies are found between similar data abstracted by the two clerks. Which data quality component is lacking?

a. Completeness
b. Validity
c. Reliability
d. Timeliness

26. According to accreditation standards, which document must be placed in the patient's record before a surgical procedure may be performed?

a. Admission record
b. Physician's order
c. Report of history and physical examination
d. Discharge summary

27. Code the following scenario: Patient admitted with major depression, recurrent, severe.

a. F33.3
b. F33.2
c. F32.9
d. F33.9

F32.9	Major depressive disorder, single episode, unspecified
F33.2	Major depressive disorder, recurrent, severe, without psychotic features
F33.3	Major depressive disorder, recurrent, severe, with psychotic symptoms
F33.9	Major depressive disorder, recurrent, unspecified

28. In ICD-10-CM this note means "not coded here":

a. Includes
b. Excludes2
c. Excludes1
d. See

29. CMS and the Joint Commission both require that healthcare professionals assess the work of colleagues in the same profession; this process is known as:

a. Peer review
b. Utilization review
c. Workflow process
d. Mediation

30. Verbal orders by telephone or in person are discouraged. For cases in which verbal orders are necessary, which of the following is the most effective method for lessening the risk of miscommunication?

   a. The person receiving the order should read it back to ensure the order is correct.
   b. The order should be signed after the patient is discharged from the facility.
   c. The order should be signed by another provider.
   d. The person receiving the order should authenticate the order after it is entered into the record.

31. The patient is 47 years old. What is the correct code for an initial inguinal herniorrhaphy for incarcerated hernia?

   a. 49496, Repair, initial inguinal hernia, full-term infant younger than age 6 months, or preterm infant older than 50 weeks postconception age and younger than age 6 months at the time of surgery, with or without hydrocelectomy; incarcerated or strangulated
   b. 49501, Repair initial inguinal hernia, age 6 months to younger than 5 years, with or without hydrocelectomy; incarcerated or strangulated
   c. 49507, Repair initial inguinal hernia, age 5 years or older; incarcerated or strangulated
   d. 49521, Repair recurrent inguinal hernia, any age; incarcerated or strangulated

32. When an entity relational diagram is implemented as a relational database, an entity will become a(n):

   a. Query
   b. Form
   c. Object
   d. Table

33. What type of health record policies dictate how long individual health records must remain available for authorized use?

   a. Disclosure policies
   b. Legal policies
   c. Retention policies
   d. Redisclosure policies

34. One of benefits of this type of data entry is that it is easy to determine if the data are complete.

   a. Big data
   b. Structured data
   c. Aggregate data
   d. Unstructured data

35. What term is used to refer to an organized collection of data that has been stored electronically to facilitate easy access?

   a. Digital formatting
   b. Database
   c. Telemedicine
   d. Data capture

36. In which EHR database model is all of the healthcare entity's patient health information stored in one system?

a. Distributed

b. Centralized

c. Hybrid

d. Traditional

37. A core data set developed by the American Society for Testing and Materials (ASTM) to communicate a patient's past and current health information as the patient transitions from one care setting to another is:

a. Continuity of care record

b. Minimum Data Set

c. Ambulatory Care Data Set

d. Uniform Hospital Discharge Data Set

38. The function that includes compiling the pertinent information from the health record, based on predetermined data sets, to enter into a separate database is called:

a. Abstracting

b. Data dictionary

c. Data migration

d. Analysis

39. A procedure that attempts to obstruct the blood flow to a malignant tumor would be coded to which root operation in ICD-10-PCS?

a. Restriction

b. Bypass

c. Occlusion

d. Dilation

40. Bob Jones is considering contractors for his company's medical benefits, and he is reviewing health plans from two different entities. Which of the following databases should he consult to compare the performance of the two health plans?

a. HEDIS

b. OASIS

c. ORYX

d. UHDDS

41. In data quality management, the process of translating data into information to be utilized by an application is called:

a. Analysis

b. Warehousing

c. Collection

d. Application

Domain 2 *Information Protection: Access, Disclosure, Archival, Privacy, and Security*

42. Copies of personal health records (PHRs) are considered part of the legal health record when:

    a. Consulted by the provider to gain information on a consumer's health history

    b. Used by the healthcare entity to provide treatment

    c. Used by the provider to obtain information on a consumer's prescription history

    d. Used by the healthcare entity to determine a consumer's DNR status

43. Under what access security mechanism would an individual be allowed access to ePHI if he or she has a proper login and password, belongs to a specified group, and his or her workstation is located in a specific place within the facility?

    a. Role-based

    b. User-based

    c. Context-based

    d. Job-based

44. Which of the following is the systematic process of identifying security measures to afford protections based on a healthcare entity's specific environment?

    a. Gap analysis

    b. Operations review

    c. Readiness assessment

    d. Risk analysis

45. What is the most common type of security threat to a health information system?

    a. External to the healthcare entity

    b. Internal to the healthcare entity

    c. Environmental in nature

    d. Computer viruses

46. Mary is contemplating triple bypass surgery. Informed consent by her surgeon would typically contain which of the following?

    a. Guarantees for outcomes

    b. Risks associated with the procedure

    c. Insurance coverage for the procedure

    d. Right to access the health record of treatment

47. Entity authentication means a computer:

    a. Prevents rebooting to deactivate a log-off system

    b. Reads a predetermined set of criteria to determine if a user is who he or she claims to be

    c. Allows rebooting to activate a sign-in process

    d. Rejects multiple log-ins

48. The security devices situated between the routers of a private network and a public network to protect the private network from unauthorized users are called:

a. Audit trails

b. Passwords

c. Firewalls

d. Encryptors

49. Which of the following is a rule established by an administrative agency of government?

a. Municipal code

b. Statute

c. Subpoena

d. Regulation

50. An inherent weakness or absence of a safeguard that could be explained by a threat is a:

a. Security incident

b. Breach

c. Vulnerability

d. Sanction

51. The computer notified the compliance officer that a user accessed the PHI of a patient with the same last name as the user. This is an example of a(n):

a. Authentication

b. Trigger

c. Transmission security

d. Integrity

52. The Security Incident Procedures Standard has one required implementation specification centered on:

a. Performing the Security Risk Analysis

b. Identifying and responding to security events

c. Preventing workforce security risks

d. Complying with breach notification processes

53. Dr. Smith, an OB-GYN specialist, has just become a staff member at Medical Center Hospital, where she may offer care and treatment related to obstetrics and gynecology including performing deliveries and gynecological surgery. The process of defining what services she may perform is called:

a. Outcomes management

b. Care mapping

c. Granting privileges

d. Retrospective review

54. Under the HIPAA privacy standard, which of the following types of protected health information (PHI) must be specifically identified in an authorization?

a. History and physical reports
b. Operative reports
c. Consultation reports
d. Psychotherapy notes

55. If a data breach caused by willful neglect is corrected within 30 days from the date of the covered entity or business associate becoming aware of it, what level of violation of the HIPAA Omnibus Rule is this breach?

a. Tier 1
b. Tier 2
c. Tier 3
d. Tier 4

56. Per the HIPAA Privacy Rule, which of the following requires authorization for research purposes?

a. Use of Mary's deidentified information about her myocardial infarction
b. Use of Mary's information about her asthma in a limited data set
c. Use of Mary's individually identifiable information related to her asthma treatments
d. Use of medical information about Jim, Mary's deceased husband

57. The Patient Self-Determination Act requires healthcare providers to:

a. Only inform patients of their right to create advance directives
b. Only document the presence or absence of an advance directive in a patient's health record
c. Write advance directives for patients who do not have them
d. Inform patients of their right to create advance directives and document the presence or absence of an advance directive in a patient's health record

58. City Hospital's HIPAA committee is considering a change in policy to allow hospital employees who are also hospital patients to access their own patient information in the hospital's EHR system. A committee member notes that HIPAA provides rights to patients to view their own health information. However, another member wonders if this action might present other problems. In this situation, what suggestion should the HIM director provide?

a. HIPAA requires that employees have access to their own information, so privileges should be granted to the employees to perform this function.
b. HIPAA does not allow employees to have access to their own information, so the policy should not be implemented.
c. Allowing employees to access their own records using their job-based access rights appears to violate HIPAA's minimum necessary requirement; therefore, allow employees to access their records through normal procedures.
d. Employees are considered a special class of people under HIPAA and the policy should be implemented.

59. Johnny is 12 years old and his parents are divorced. In order for Johnny to receive medical treatment, generally:

a. Both parents must consent

b. One parent must consent

c. A court-appointed guardian must consent

d. Johnny can consent

60. This process provides covered entities and business associates with the structural framework upon which to build their HIPAA Security Plan.

a. Security Rule Evaluation

b. Security Rule Assessment

c. Security Incident Analysis

d. Security Risk Analysis

61. The Information Access Management Standard specifically requires that healthcare entities include specifications around:

a. Controlling access to a workstation, transaction, program, or process

b. Providing workforce security

c. Establishing procedures for workforce access

d. Assessing security measures

62. An employee forgot his user ID badge at home and uses another employee's badge to access the computer system. What controls should have been in place to minimize this security breach?

a. Access controls

b. Security incident procedures

c. Security management process

d. Workforce security awareness training

63. The process of releasing health record documentation originally created by a different provider is called:

a. Privileged communication

b. Subpoena

c. Jurisdiction

d. Redisclosure

64. Today, Janet Kim had her first appointment with a new dentist. She was not presented with a Notice of Privacy Practices. Is this acceptable?

a. No, a dentist is a healthcare clearinghouse, which is a covered entity under HIPAA.

b. Yes, a dentist is not a covered entity per the HIPAA Privacy Rule.

c. No, it is a violation of the HIPAA Privacy Rule.

d. Yes, the Notice of Privacy Practices is not required.

65. Mercy Hospital personnel need to review the health records of Katie Grace for utilization review purposes (#1). They will also be sending her records to her physician for continuity of care (#2). Under HIPAA, these two functions are:

   a. Use (#1) and disclosure (#2)
   b. Request (#1) and disclosure (#2)
   c. Disclosure (#1) and use (#2)
   d. Disclosures (#1 and #2)

66. Jennifer's widowed mother is elderly and often confused. She has asked Jennifer to accompany her to physician office visits because she often forgets to tell the physician vital information. Under the Privacy Rule, the release of her mother's PHI to Jennifer is:

   a. Never allowed
   b. Allowed when the information is directly relevant to Jennifer's involvement in her mother's care or treatment
   c. Allowed only if Jennifer's mother is declared incompetent by a court of law
   d. Allowed access to PHI; any family member is always allowed access to PHI

67. The "custodian of health records" refers to the individual within a healthcare entity who is responsible for which of the following actions?

   a. Determining alternative treatment for the patient
   b. Preparing physicians to testify
   c. Testifying to the authenticity of records
   d. Testifying regarding the care of the patient

68. Regarding life-sustaining treatment and a patient's right of self-determination, courts have generally held that:

   a. A competent adult does not have the right to refuse medical treatment.
   b. A competent adult gives up the right to refuse medical treatment if the physician believes the refusal is morally wrong.
   c. An incompetent adult has a right to the withdrawal of medical treatment if that incompetent adult, while competent, expressed his or her wishes and the state now determines that the evidence of those wishes is sufficient.
   d. A competent adult cannot make healthcare decisions based on his or her religious beliefs.

69. Champion Hospital retains Hall and Hall, a law firm, to perform all of its legal work, including representation during medical malpractice lawsuits. Which of the following statements is correct?

   a. The law firm is not a business associate because it is a legal, not a medical, organization.
   b. The law firm is a business associate because it performs activities on behalf of the hospital.
   c. The law firm is not a business associate because the privacy rule prohibits it from using individually identifiable information.
   d. The law firm is not a business associate because it is a medical, not a legal, organization.

70. A visitor walks through the work area and picks up a flash drive from an employee's desk. What security controls should have been implemented to prevent this security breach?

a. Device and media controls

b. Facility access controls

c. Workstation use controls

d. Workstation security controls

71. On review of the audit trail for an EHR system, the HIM director discovers that a departmental employee with authorized access to patient records is printing far more records than the average user. In this case, what should the supervisor do?

a. Reprimand the employee

b. Fire the employee

c. Determine what information was printed and why

d. Revoke the employee's access privileges

72. A hospital is planning on allowing coding professionals to work at home. The hospital is in the process of identifying strategies to minimize the security risks associated with this practice. Which of the following would be best to ensure that data breaches are minimized when the home computer is unattended?

a. User name and password

b. Automatic session terminations

c. Cable locks

d. Encryption

73. The medical staff at Regency Health is nationally renowned for its skill in performing cardiac procedures. The nursing staff in the cardiac unit has noticed that a significant number of health records do not have informed consents prior to the performance of procedures. Obtaining informed consent is the responsibility of the:

a. Nursing staff

b. Admissions department

c. Physician

d. Administration

74. Susan is completing her required high school community service hours by serving as a volunteer at the local hospital. Relative to the hospital, Susan is a(n):

a. Business associate

b. Employee

c. Workforce member

d. Covered entity

75. Jeremy Lykins was required to undergo a physical exam prior to becoming employed by San Fernando Hospital. Jeremy's medical information is:

a. Protected by the Privacy Rule because it is individually identifiable

b. Not protected by the Privacy Rule because it is part of a personnel record

c. Protected by the Privacy Rule because it contains his physical exam results

d. Protected by the Privacy Rule because it is in the custody of a covered entity

76. What is the other term used to denote contingency planning required by HIPAA?

    a. Data backup
    b. Data recovery
    c. Disaster recovery planning
    d. Emergency mode of operation

77. The original HIPAA legislation required adoption of four identifiers: employers, providers, health plans, and individuals. Three of these identifiers have been implemented and one is on hold. Which unique identifier has ***not*** been implemented?

    a. Employers
    b. Health plans
    c. Individuals
    d. Providers

78. Shirley Denton has written to request an amendment of her PHI from Bon Voyage Hospital, stating that incorrect information is present on the document in question. The document is an incident report from Bon Voyage Hospital that was erroneously placed in Ms. Denton's health record. The covered entity declines to grant her request based on which Privacy Rule provision?

    a. It was not created by the covered entity.
    b. It is not part of the designated record set.
    c. None; the covered entity must grant her request.
    d. Her attending physician did not authorize the amendment.

79. Community Hospital is discussing restricting the access that physicians have to electronic clinical records. The medical record committee is divided on how to approach this issue. Some committee members maintain that all information should be available; whereas, others maintain that HIPAA restricts access. The HIM director is part of the committee. Which of the following statements should the director advise to the committee?

    a. HIPAA restricts physician access to all information.
    b. The "minimum necessary" concept does not apply to disclosures made for treatment purposes; therefore, physician access should not be restricted.
    c. The "minimum necessary" concept does not apply to disclosures made for treatment purposes, but the healthcare entity must define what physicians need as part of their treatment role.
    d. The "minimum necessary" concept applies only to attending physician; therefore, restriction of access must be implemented.

80. The HIM supervisor suspects that a departmental employee is accessing the EHR for personal reasons but has no specific data to support this suspicion. In this case, what should the supervisor do?

    a. Confront the employee.
    b. Send out a memorandum to all department employees reminding them of the hospital's policy on Internet use.
    c. Ask the security officer for audit trail data to confirm or disprove the suspicion.
    d. Transfer the employee to another job that does not require computer usage.

81. Protected health information that is maintained in a designated record set can be accessed by the patient or other authorized party upon request. Covered entities must respond to requests within what timeframe after receipt of the request?

a. 15 days
b. 30 days
c. 60 days
d. 90 days

82. If a patient has health insurance but pays in full for a healthcare service and asks that the information be kept private, under HIPAA the covered entity must:

a. Release the information to the health insurance provider
b. Get special patient consent to release the information
c. Comply with the patient's request and keep the information private
d. Request permission from HHS to release the information

83. One of the medical staff committees at St. Vincent Hospital is responsible for reviewing cases of patients readmitted within 14 days after discharge. This review of the patients' health records is considered healthcare:

a. Actions
b. Operations
c. Payment
d. Treatment

84. An EHR system can provide better security than a paper record system for protected health information due to:

a. Handling by fewer clinical practitioners
b. Access controls, audit trails, and authentication systems
c. Easier data entry
d. Safer storage

85. A hospital receives a valid request from a patient for copies of her medical records. The HIM clerk who is preparing the records removes copies of the patient's records from another hospital where the patient was previously treated. According to HIPAA regulations, was this action correct?

a. Yes, HIPAA only requires that current records be produced for the patient.
b. Yes, this is hospital policy over which HIPAA has no control.
c. No, the records from the previous hospital are considered to be included in the designated record set and should be given to the patient.
d. No, the records from the previous hospital are not included in the designated record set but should be released anyway.

86. The Person or Entity Authentication Standard requires methods for verifying that a person is who he or she claims to be. Any of the following meets this standard ***except***:

a. Biometrics
b. Smart card
c. Unit level password
d. Physical token

Domain 3 *Informatics, Analytics, and Data Use*

87. The computer-based process of extracting, quantifying, and filtering data that reside in a database is called:
    a. Autocoding
    b. Bar coding
    c. Data mining
    d. Intelligent character recognition

88. Working with the healthcare entity's integration team to ensure that ADT interfaces are properly built and tested is the responsibility of the:
    a. MPI manager
    b. EHR analyst
    c. IT manager
    d. Electronic forms manager

89. To be successful, any information system tactical plan must align with:
    a. Current hardware in use in the facility
    b. The healthcare entity's strategic plan
    c. IS department strategies
    d. Health information management initiatives

90. In which of the following examples does the gender of the patient constitute information rather than a data element?
    a. As an entry to be completed on the face sheet of the health record
    b. In the note "50-year-old white male" in the patient history
    c. In a study comparing the incidence of myocardial infarctions in black males as compared to white females
    d. In a study of the age distribution of lung cancer patients

91. Which of the following examples illustrates data that have been transformed into meaningful information?
    a. 45 percent
    b. 3,567 units of penicillin
    c. $5 million saved
    d. Average length of stay at Holt Hospital is 5.6 days

92. Which of the following allows a patient to access all or part of the health record that is maintained by the provider?
    a. Clinical decision support
    b. Digital dictation
    c. Patient portal
    d. WebMD

93. The distribution in this curve is:

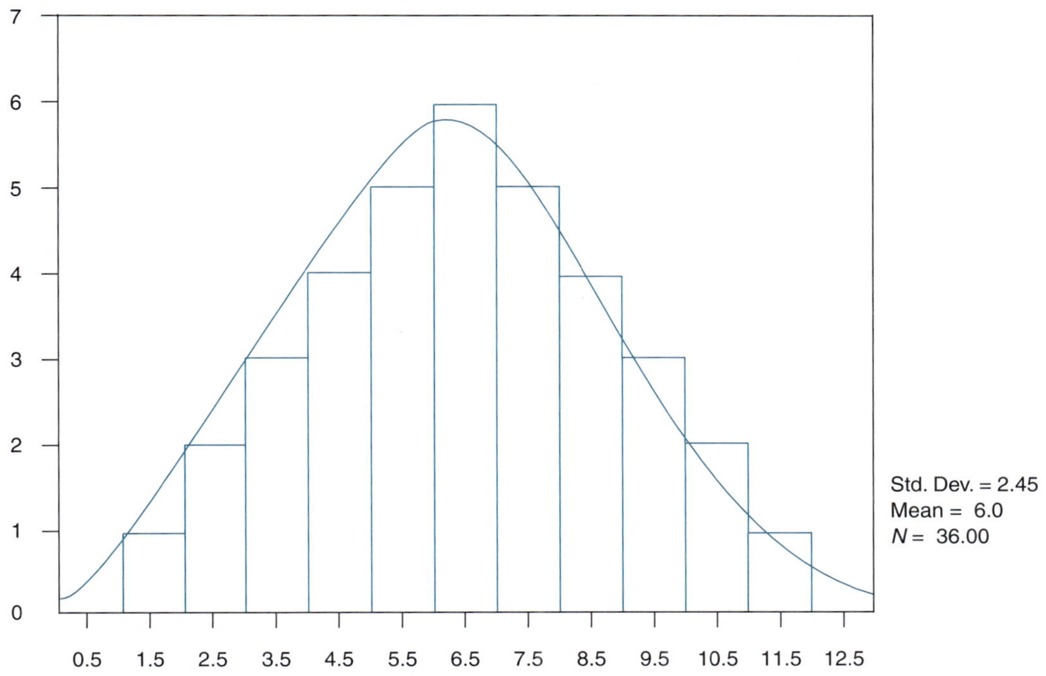

a. Skewed left
b. Bimodal
c. Normal
d. Skewed right

94. Dr. Smith orders 500 mg of penicillin by mouth three times a day for Jane Doe, who is being seen in the hospital emergency department. The computer sends an alert to Dr. Smith to tell her the patient, Jane Doe, is allergic to penicillin. What type of computer system is Dr. Smith using?

a. Clinical data repository
b. Data exchange standard
c. Clinical decision support
d. Health informatics standard

95. You want to graph the number of deaths due to prostate cancer from 2010 through 2017. Which graphic tool would you use?

a. Frequency polygon
b. Histogram
c. Line graph or plot
d. Pie chart

96. The director of the health information department wanted to determine the level of physicians' satisfaction with the department's services. The director surveyed the physicians who came to the department. What type of sample is this?

a. Direct

b. Positive

c. Guided

d. Convenience

97. After evaluating the following graph, what information can be determined from these data?

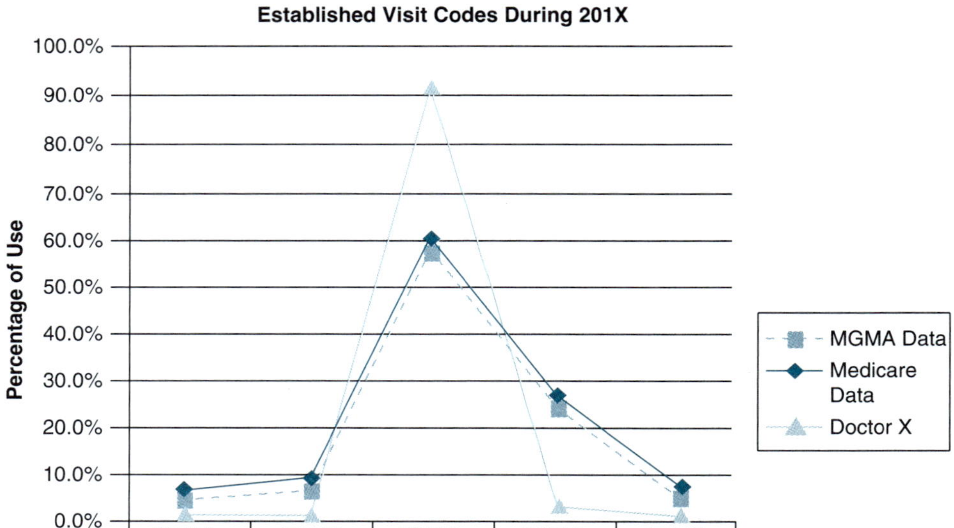

	99211	99212	99213	99214	99215
MGMA Data	3.5%	9.7%	60.6%	22.4%	3.8%
Medicare Data	4.7%	9.2%	59.5%	22.6%	4.1%
Doctor X	3.0%	1.0%	92.0%	4.0%	0.0%

a. Doctor X uses code 99215 less frequently than his peers.

b. Doctor X's documentation doesn't support the codes submitted.

c. Doctor X overutilizes code 99213 as compared with the documentation.

d. Doctor X overutilizes code 99212 as compared with his peers.

98. The MPI includes which of the following?

a. Patient's date of birth, height, and gender

b. Patient's health record number, blood pressure reading, and age

c. Patient's gender, height, and weight

d. Patient's date of birth, gender, and health record number

99. Using the admission criteria provided, determine if the following patient meets severity of illness and intensity of service criteria for admission.

Severity of Illness	Intensity of Service
Persistent fever	Inpatient-approved surgery or procedure within 24 hours of admission
Active bleeding	Intravenous medications or fluid replacement
Wound dehiscence	Vital signs every 2 hours or more often

John Smith presents to the emergency room at 1500 hours with a fever of 101 degrees F, which he has had for the last three days. He was discharged six days ago following a colon resection. X-rays show a bowel obstruction and the plan is to admit him to surgery in the morning.

a. The patient does not meet both severity of illness and intensity of service criteria.

b. The patient does meet both severity of illness and intensity of service criteria.

c. The patient meets intensity of service criteria but not severity of illness criteria.

d. The patient meets severity of illness criteria but not intensity of service criteria.

100. This type of data display tool is a plotted chart of data that shows the progress of a process over time.

a. Bar graph

b. Histogram

c. Pie chart

d. Line graph or plot

101. The integrity of the MPI is key to accurate storage and retrieval of patient-related information. Errors are possible in the MPI for various reasons. Errors in the MPI database can lead to which of the following?

a. Billing problems

b. Accurate record location

c. Necessary patient testing

d. Efficiency in the HIM department

102. In purchasing an EHR system from a vendor, what does due diligence refer to?

a. Checking references

b. Conducting product demonstrations

c. Financing the investment

d. Negotiating the contract

103. A hospital is undergoing a major reconstruction project and a new director of nursing has been hired. At the same time, the nursing documentation component of the EHR has been implemented. The fact that nursing staff satisfaction scores have risen is:

a. A result of anecdotal benefits of EHR

b. A result of qualitative benefits of EHR

c. A result of reconfiguration of the nursing units

d. Uncertain due to existence of confounding variables

104. Using the data in the following graph, we can see changes in this hospital's profile. What concerns might the hospital's quality council need to address based on these changes in their customer base?

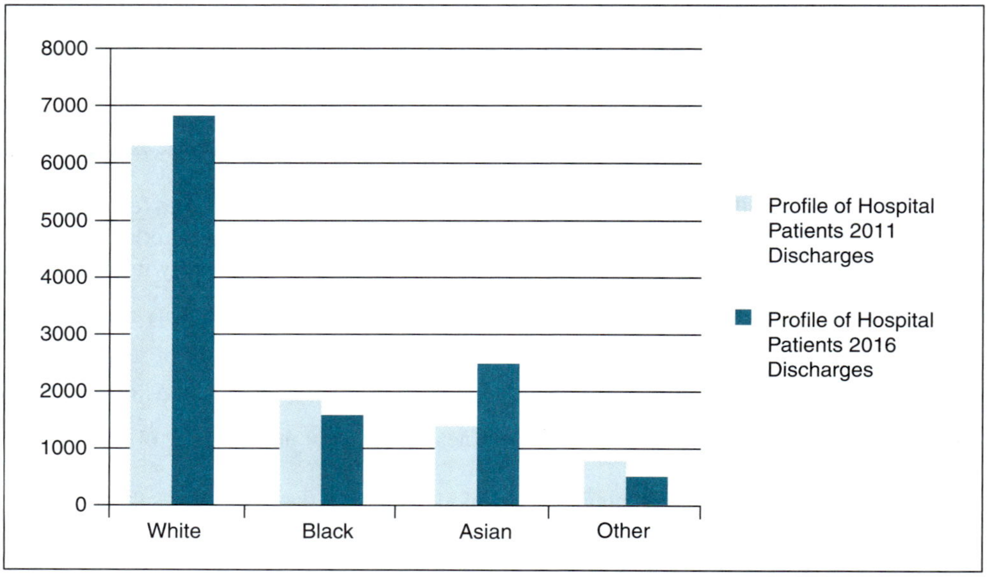

a. Staffing changes might be necessary to accommodate patients who have cultural differences.

b. Data collection has improved.

c. No changes in staffing are necessary because the patient mix is appropriate.

d. The quality council should ask for more detailed data.

105. There were 25 inpatient deaths, including newborns, at Community Memorial Hospital during the month of June. The hospital performed five autopsies during the same period. The gross autopsy rate for the hospital for June was:

a. 0.02%

b. 0.2%

c. 5%

d. 20%

106. Which of the following represents the correct sequence (from low to high) of levels of interoperability?

a. Semantic, basic, functional

b. Basic, functional, semantic

c. Functional, process, semantic

d. Functional, semantic, basic

107. Community Memorial Hospital discharged nine patients on April 1st. The length of stay for each patient is shown in the following table. What is the mode length of stay for this group of patients?

Patient	Number of Days
A	1
B	5
C	3
D	3
E	8
F	8
G	8
H	9
I	9

a. 5 days
b. 6 days
c. 8 days
d. 9 days

108. If an analyst wishes to determine the root cause of claim denials during June via a random sample, what is the sampling unit?

a. Patient
b. Hospital
c. Claim
d. Payer

109. In which stage of the system life cycle would data be collected from system users regarding their needs?

a. Implementation
b. Design
c. Analysis
d. Initiation

110. What is the biggest problem with using mean length of stay as a facility statistic?

a. It is not accurate.
b. It is influenced by outlier values.
c. It is mathematically incorrect.
d. It is a dependent variable.

111. What architectural model of health information exchange allows participants to access data in point-to-point exchange?

a. Consolidated
b. Federated—consistent databases
c. Federated—inconsistent databases
d. Switch

112. Which of the following basic services provided by an HIE entity ensures that information can be retrieved as needed?

a. Consent management
b. Person identification
c. Registry and directory
d. Secure data transport

113. Using the following data, what conclusions can you draw about Dr. Jones's outcomes compared to the OB/GYN practice group?

Category	Dr. Jones	OB/GYN Group
Cesarean section rate	15.2%	11.5%
Hospital-acquired infection	1.7%	1.5%
Surgical wound infection rate	3.8%	0.36%
Mortality rate	0.57%	0.07%

a. Dr. Jones performed better than the OB/GYN group in all four categories.
b. Dr. Jones performed poorer than the OB/GYN group in all four categories.
c. Dr. Jones performed better than the OB/GYN group in all categories except mortality rate.
d. Dr. Jones performed poorer than the OB/GYN group in all categories except the mortality rate.

114. Which of the following health record numbers are in correct terminal digit order?

a. 00-52-84, 07-48-81, 45-58-81, 65-59-87
b. 12-25-62, 11-25-68, 18-20-69, 00-24-69
c. 01-52-25, 02-53-25, 03-22-35, 35-20-35
d. 00-01-10, 52-01-11, 26-00-00, 00-00-12

115. As a preliminary step in designing an IS strategy, it is important for the steering committee to conduct a scan of the external environment and to:

a. Build security and privacy constraints
b. Contact vendors for system bids
c. Purchase hardware and software components
d. Conduct an internal environmental assessment

116. Which request for proposal (RFP) component would fit the following description: Describe how your product supports the ability to register a patient in the clinic, admit the patient using the same health record number and demographic information, and share the medication list for medication reconciliation with the nursing home to which the patient is discharged.

a. Application support
b. Operational requirements
c. Technical specifications
d. Use case

117. The key to an effective retention and retrieval system of health records in a facility is:

a. Master patient index

b. Terminal digit filing

c. Microfilm

d. Optical imaging

118. Which of the following would be used to determine what the users need in an information system?

a. Questionnaire

b. Trouble ticket

c. Source code

d. Weighted system

119. Which of the following indexes and databases includes patient-identifiable information?

a. MEDLINE

b. Clinical trials database

c. Master population/patient index

d. UMLS

120. Which of the following is an effective method of evaluating responses to a request for proposal (RFP)?

a. Testing the new system

b. Negotiating contracts with all vendors and assessing the best price

c. Attending user group meetings

d. Visiting sites that use the systems of product competitors

121. Online or real-time transaction processing (OLTP) is a functional requirement for a:

a. Data repository

b. Data mart

c. Data display

d. Data dictionary

122. Barcoding technology is an example of:

a. Automatic recognition technology

b. Artificial intelligence

c. Voice recognition

d. Vector graphic data

123. Physicians use the ________ to access multiple sources of patient information within the healthcare organization's network.

a. Data repository

b. Clinical information system

c. Data warehouse

d. Clinician portal

124. HIPAA mandated that healthcare business partners and covered entities implement a common standard for data and information transfer. That standard is:

a. ICD-10-CM
b. HL7
c. ASC X12 N
d. CPT

125. Which data collection program is the basis for the CMS value-based purchasing program?

a. Leapfrog
b. HEDIS
c. Hospital Compare
d. HCUP

126. Which of the following is included in a request for proposal (RFP)?

a. Preparing and training managers
b. General product information
c. Establishing an IT infrastructure
d. The timeline for implementation

127. Which graph is the best choice to use when comparing lengths of stay across three hospitals?

a. Line graph
b. Bar chart
c. Pie chart
d. Scatter diagram

128. This analytic technique is being used by CMS to assist in prepayment audits?

a. Descriptive statistics
b. Graphical analysis
c. Exploratory data analysis
d. Predictive modeling

129. The relationship between patient gender and readmission to the hospital is best displayed using a:

a. Frequency chart
b. Contingency table
c. Bar chart
d. Pie chart

Domain 4 *Revenue Management*

130. A coding supervisor audits coded records to ensure the codes reflect the actual documentation in the health record. This coding auditing process addresses the data quality element of:

a. Granularity

b. Reliability

c. Timeliness

d. Accuracy

131. The term "hard coding" refers to:

a. ICD-10-CM codes that are coded by the coders

b. CPT codes that appear in the hospital's chargemaster

c. CPT codes that are coded by the coders

d. ICD-10-CM codes that appear in the hospital's chargemaster

132. Which type of identity theft occurs when a patient uses another person's name and insurance information to receive healthcare benefits?

a. Criminal

b. Financial

c. Health

d. Medical

133. A coding audit shows that an inpatient coder is using multiple codes that describe the individual components of a procedure rather than using a single code that describes all the steps of the procedure performed. Which of the following should be done in this case?

a. Require all coders to implement this practice

b. Report the practice to the OIG

c. Counsel the coder to stop the practice immediately

d. Put the coder on an unpaid leave of absence

134. In developing a coding compliance program, which of the following would ***not*** be ordinarily included as participants in coding compliance education?

a. Current coding personnel

b. Medical staff

c. Newly hired coding personnel

d. Nursing staff

135. Aging of accounts is the practice of counting the days, generally in increments, from the time a bill has been sent to the payer to the current day. What is the standard increment, in days, that most healthcare entities use for the aging of accounts?

a. 7-day increment

b. 14-day increment

c. 30-day increment

d. 90-day increment

136. What is the benefit of comparing the coding assigned by coders to the coding that appears on the claim?

a. May find that more codes are required to support the claim
b. May find that the charge description master soft coding is inaccurate
c. Serves as a way for HIM to take over the management of patient financial services
d. May find claim generation issues that cannot be found in other ways

137. When documentation in the health record is not clear, the coding professional should:

a. Query the physician who originated the progress note or other report in question
b. Refer to dictation from other encounters with the patient to get clarification
c. Submit the question to the coding clinic
d. Query a physician who consistently responds to queries in a timely manner

138. Using the information provided, if this is a participating physician who accepts assignment, how much can he or she expect to be reimbursed by Medicare?

> Physician's normal charge = $340
> Medicare fee schedule = $300
> Patient has met his deductible

a. $140
b. $240
c. $300
d. $340

139. Which of the following lists contains only entities that have roles in the various Medicare Improper Payment Review processes?

a. MAC, RAC, and QIO
b. AMA, AHA, and RAC
c. MAC, AMA, and QIO
d. ACS, MAC, and RAC

140. Which of the following is the definition of revenue cycle management?

a. The regularly repeating set of events that produce revenue or income
b. The method by which patients are grouped together based on a set of characteristics
c. The systematic comparison of the products, services, and outcomes of one healthcare entity with those of a similar entity
d. The coordination of all administrative and clinical functions that contribute to the capture, management, and collection of patient service revenue

141. Which of the following accreditation categories would the Joint Commission assign to a hospital that did not meet all of the standards at the time of the initial on-site survey, had a level of standards in noncompliance, had Requirements for Improvements (RFIs) in excess of the published level for the year, and subsequently underwent an additional on-site, follow-up survey?

a. Accreditation with follow-up survey

b. Preliminary accreditation

c. Accredited

d. Contingent accreditation

142. The most recent coding audit has revealed a tendency to miss secondary diagnoses that would have increased the reimbursement for the case. Which of the following strategies will help to identify and correct these cases in the short term?

a. Focus reviews on lower-weighted MS-DRGs from triples and pairs

b. Identify the facility's top 10 to 15 APCs by volume and charges

c. Contract with a larger consulting firm to do audits and education

d. Focus reviews on surgical complications

143. The Civilian Health and Medical Program of the Department of Veterans Affairs (CHAMPVA) is available for:

a. Veterans of the Armed Forces

b. Spouses or widow(er)s of veterans meeting specific criteria

c. Active-duty service members

d. Spouses of active-duty service members

144. When the physician does not specify the method used to remove a lesion during an endoscopy, what action should the coder take?

a. Assign the removal by snare technique code

b. Assign the removal by hot biopsy forceps code

c. Assign the ablation code

d. Query the physician as to the method used

145. During the voluntary review process, the performance of a healthcare entity is measured against:

a. Accreditation standards

b. Clinical practice guidelines

c. Core measures

d. Conditions of Participation

146. After a claim has been filed with Medicare, a healthcare entity had late charges posted to a patient's outpatient account that changed the calculation of the ambulatory payment classification (APC). What is the best practice for this entity to receive the correct reimbursement from Medicare?

a. Nothing, because the claim has already been submitted

b. Bill the patient for any remaining balance after payment from Medicare is received

c. Submit an adjusted claim to Medicare

d. Return the account to coding for review

147. Most facilities begin counting days in accounts receivable at which of the following times?

a. Date the patient registers
b. Date the patient is discharged
c. Date the claim drops
d. Date the claim is received by the payer

148. What type of organization works under contract with CMS to conduct Medicare and Medicaid certification surveys for hospitals?

a. Accreditation organizations
b. Certification organizations
c. State licensure agencies
d. Conditions of Participation agencies

149. All of the following are goals for a clinical documentation improvement program ***except***:

a. Promoting record completion during the patient's stay
b. Identifying missing, conflicting, or nonspecific documentation
c. Improving communication between the physician and the care team
d. Preventing billing for bundled services

150. A polyp was removed from a patient's colon during a colonoscopy procedure. The physician and pathologist document the polyp as probable adenocarcinoma of the colon. Which of the following actions should the coding professional take to code this encounter?

a. Code "polyp"
b. Code "adenoma of the colon"
c. Code "adenocarcinoma of the colon"
d. Query the physician

151. The facility's Medicare case-mix index has dropped, although other statistical measures appear constant. The CFO suspects coding errors. What type of coding audit review should be performed?

a. Random audit
b. Focused audit
c. Compliance audit
d. External audit

152. A comprehensive retrospective review should be conducted at least once a year of what aspect of the CDI program?

a. Proficiency statistics
b. Compliance issues
c. All query opportunities
d. Core key measures

153. The physician's office sent a request for payment to Able Insurance Company. The term used in the healthcare industry for this request for payment is a(n):

a. Allowance

b. Reimbursement

c. Block grant

d. Claim

Domain 5 *Leadership*

154. The process of conducting a thorough review of the internal and external conditions in which a healthcare entity operates is called:

a. Environmental assessment

b. Operations improvement planning

c. Strategic management

d. Employment assessment

155. What term is used to represent a difference between the budgeted amount and the actual amount of a line item that is not expected to reverse itself during a subsequent period?

a. Permanent variance

b. Fixed cost

c. Temporary variance

d. Flexible cost

156. According to the records kept on filing unit performance over the past year, the filing unit has filed an average of 1,000 records per day. There are three full-time equivalent (FTE) record filers in the department who are productive 88 percent of each workday (that is, 12 percent unproductive or 12 percent PFD). Based on this information, the average number of records filed per productive hour per FTE is:

a. 14 records per hour

b. 16 records per hour

c. 37 records per hour

d. 48 records per hour

157. Successful strategic managers understand that three competencies are common to all successful change and that these competencies can and must be developed. These three competencies are:

a. Leadership, change management, and strategic development

b. Organizational learning, visioning, and leadership

c. Visioning, managing, and change management

d. Improvement, visioning, and managing

158. In order to expedite basic performance improvement team functioning, the team should:

a. Use unstructured brainstorming

b. Perform force field analysis

c. Establish ground rules

d. Use structured brainstorming

159. Identifying future health information needs for a healthcare entity and projecting specific initiatives required to meet those needs is part of:

a. Data modeling

b. Policy development

c. Strategic planning

d. Workflow modeling

160. Outpatient programs designed to provide employees immediate access to psychological counseling on a limited basis that may be provided on-site or through local providers are called:

a. Health benefits fair

b. Employee assistance programs

c. Outpatient employee care

d. Employee crisis lines

161. Which discipline defines the natural laws of work and focuses on employee comfort and safety?

a. Aesthetics

b. Cybernetics

c. Affinity grouping

d. Ergonomics

162. The process icon symbol 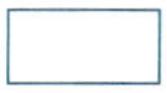 is used in flowcharting to indicate:

a. A process in which actions are being performed by humans

b. A point in the process at which participants must evaluate the status of the process

c. Formal procedures that participants are expected to carry out the same way every time

d. A point in the process at which the participants must record data in paper-based or computer-based formats

163. Which of the following is most important in securing support for a change program?

a. Understanding that individuals accept change in their own way

b. Clear directives from senior management

c. Assurances that no one will lose his or her job

d. Being clear about the rewards for those who are on board

164. Which of the following is a conflict management method in which both parties meet with an objective third party to explore their perceptions and feelings?

a. Compromise

b. Collaborative confrontation

c. Control

d. Constructive confrontation

165. The Hay method is used to measure the three levels of major compensable factors: the know-how, problem-solving, and accountability requirements of each position. This system is used for:

a. Job evaluation

b. Interviewing applicants

c. Performance measurement

d. Work scheduling

166. For a contract to be valid, it must include three elements. Which of the following is one of those elements?

a. Assumption of risk

b. Consideration

c. Statute of limitations

d. Notice of liability

167. The performance standard to "assign the correct health record number to a returning patient with 99 percent accuracy" is an example of a:

a. Compliance standard

b. Quantity standard

c. Joint Commission standard

d. Quality standard

168. Distributing work duties to others along with the right to make decisions and take action is called:

a. Accountability

b. Coaching

c. Delegation

d. Communication

169. Monitoring risks during the project management process is important because:

a. The work breakdown structure is hierarchical, not necessarily chronological.

b. After the initial planning is complete, no changes to the schedule are needed.

c. The project team members need a list of tasks to perform.

d. Minor changes to the scope of the project can turn into more significant changes to the original work or cost estimates.

Use the following information to answer questions 170 and 171.

Triad Healthcare Financial Data 12/31/201X	
Cash	$500,000
A/R	$250,000
Building	$1,000,000
Land	$700,000
A/P	$350,000
Mortgage	$600,000
Revenue	$2,500,000
Expenses	$2,250,000

170. Based on the financial data listed above, what was Triad's net income?

a. $150,000

b. $250,000

c. $400,000

d. $1,500,000

171. Based on the financial data listed, what was Triad's total net assets before posting net income for the year?

a. $250,000

b. $400,000

c. $1,250,000

d. $1,500,000

172. At a cost of $12,000, Community Hospital is refinancing the mortgage on the building that houses its clinic. The hospital will save $500 a month in interest. What is the payback period on the refinancing?

a. 15 months

b. 18 months

c. 1 year

d. 2 years

173. Fifty percent of an HIM department's staff have a nationally recognized credential. This is an example of what type of performance measurement:

a. System

b. Process

c. Internal

d. Outcome

174. The Health Information Services department at Medical Center Hospital has identified problems with its work processes. Too much time is spent on unimportant tasks, there is duplication of effort, and task assignment is uneven in quality and volume among employees. The manager has each employee complete a form identifying the amount of time he or she spends each day on various tasks. What is this tool called?

a. Serial work distribution tool

b. Work distribution chart

c. Check sheet

d. Flow process chart

175. As an EHR implementation project proceeds, additional hospital departments add requirements for the system, and the project becomes more complex. This is known as:

a. Unaligned parameters

b. Alternative goals

c. Risk assumption

d. Scope creep

176. A distance learning method in which groups of employees in multiple classroom locations may listen to and see the material presented at the same time via satellite or telephone is called:

a. Audio conferencing

b. Computer-based training

c. Videoconferencing

d. Online learning

177. An HIM professional who accurately reports HIV status and the true results of an audit that indicates health problems meets the ethical standards for:

a. E-health

b. Integrated delivery systems

c. Public health

d. Managed care

178. Research on emotional intelligence shows that:

a. Emotions do not have much of a role in the workplace

b. A combination of feelings and rationality make managers more successful

c. It is a clearly defined measure that can be precisely assessed

d. Effective managers and successful managers are the same

179. The lead coder in a health information department has been the acknowledged coding expert for a number of years. As implementation of an computer-assisted coding (CAC) system moves forward, it becomes evident this coder has an aversion to technology, is resistant to the CAC system, and is losing confidence in her coding skills. In project management terms, this creates a:

a. Project risk

b. Technical risk

c. Failure mode

d. Scope creep

180. A large hospital is planning for an EHR but wants to ensure it has adequate source systems in place to support it. Each of the ancillary departments has a separate information system, and each has claimed that the product is the best on the market and that the vendor has promised the system will interface with any EHR on the market. Identify the project management mistake in this situation.

a. Lack of priority

b. Lack of sponsorship

c. Lack of project manager software

d. Lack of project management

PRACTICE QUESTIONS

Domain 1 Data Content, Structure, and Standards

1. A patient has HIV with disseminated candidiasis. What is the correct code assignment?

B20	Human immunodeficiency virus [HIV] disease
B37.0	Candidal stomatitis Oral thrush
B37.7	Candidal sepsis Disseminated candidiasis Systemic candidiasis
B37.89	Other sites of candidiasis Candidal osteomyelitis

a. B20, B37.0
b. B37.7, B20
c. B20, B37.7
d. B20, B37.89, B37.7

2. What term is used in reference to raw facts generally stored as characters, words, symbols, measurements, or statistics?

a. Data
b. Information
c. Knowledge
d. Notices

3. Which type of data consists of factual details aggregated or summarized from a group of health records that provides no means to identify specific patients?

a. Original
b. Source
c. Protected
d. Derived

4. What term refers to information that provides physicians with pertinent health information beyond the health record itself used to determine treatment options?

a. Core measures
b. Enhanced discharge planning
c. Data mining
d. Clinical practice guidelines

5. When a healthcare entity destroys health records after the acceptable retention period has been met, a certificate of destruction is created. How long must the healthcare entity maintain the certificate of destruction?

a. Two years
b. Five years
c. Ten years
d. Permanently

6. A patient was admitted for removal of the left lobe of the liver via laparotomy due to metastasis from a colon carcinoma. What is the correct ICD-10-PCS procedure code for this operation?

Section	Body System	Root Operation	Body Part	Approach	Device	Qualifier
Medical and Surgical	Hepatobiliary System and Pancreas	Excision	Liver, Left Lobe	Open	No Device	No Qualifier
0	F	B	2	0	Z	Z

Section	Body System	Root Operation	Body Part	Approach	Device	Qualifier
Medical and Surgical	Hepatobiliary System and Pancreas	Excision	Liver, Left Lobe	Percutaneous Endoscopic	No Device	No Qualifier
0	F	B	2	4	Z	Z

Section	Body System	Root Operation	Body Part	Approach	Device	Qualifier
Medical and Surgical	Hepatobiliary System and Pancreas	Resection	Liver, Left Lobe	Open	No Device	No Qualifier
0	F	T	2	0	Z	Z

Section	Body System	Root Operation	Body Part	Approach	Device	Qualifier
Medical and Surgical	Hepatobiliary System and Pancreas	Resection	Liver, Left Lobe	Percutaneous Endoscopic	No Device	No Qualifier
0	F	T	2	4	Z	Z

a. 0FB20ZZ
b. 0FB24ZZ
c. 0FT20ZZ
d. 0FT24ZZ

7. A 65-year-old woman was admitted to the hospital. She was diagnosed with sepsis secondary to methicillin susceptible *Staphylococcus aureus* and abdominal pain secondary to diverticulitis of the colon. What is the correct code assignment?

A41.01	Sepsis due to Methicillin susceptible *Staphylococcus aureus*
A41.89	Other specified sepsis
41.9	Sepsis, unspecified organism
B95.61	Methicillin susceptible *Staphylococcus aureus* infection as the cause of diseases classified elsewhere
K57.32	Diverticulitis of large intestine without perforation or abscess without bleeding
R10.9	Unspecified abdominal pain

a. A41.89, K57.32, R10.9
b. A41.01, K57.32
c. A41.89, K57.32, B95.61
d. A41.9, K57.32

8. A patient was admitted to the hospital and diagnosed with Type 1 diabetic gangrene. What is the correct code assignment?

E08.52	Diabetes mellitus due to underlying condition with diabetic peripheral angiopathy with gangrene
E10.52	Type 1 diabetes mellitus with diabetic peripheral angiopathy with gangrene
E10.8	Type 1 diabetes mellitus with unspecified complications
I96	Gangrene, not elsewhere classified

a. E08.52, I96
b. E10.52, I96
c. E10.8
d. E10.52

9. The patient has a biopsy of the colon followed by a hemicolectomy. In the ICD-10-PCS coding system, which procedure(s) are coded?

a. The hemicolectomy only
b. The biopsy only
c. Both the biopsy and the hemicolectomy
d. It depends on the results of the biopsy

10. Of the following, what is the most likely to happen to the health records of a physician's patient when that physician leaves an office practice?

a. It will be sent to the state department of health.
b. It will be sent to outside storage.
c. It will be destroyed.
d. It will be retained by the practice.

11. What is the first step a healthcare entity should take when developing a data dictionary?

a. Develop an approvals process
b. Integrate common data elements
c. Design a plan
d. Ensure consistency

12. Name of element, definition, application in which the data element is found, locator key, ownership, entity relationships, date first entered system, date element terminated from system, and system of origin are all examples of:

a. Autoauthentication fields
b. Metadata
c. Data
d. Information fields

13. Which of the following processes is an ancillary function of the health record?

    a. Admitting and registration information
    b. Billing and reimbursement
    c. Patient assessment and care planning
    d. Biomedical research

14. What are LOINC codes used for?

    a. Identifying test results
    b. Reporting test results
    c. Identifying tests unique to a specific company
    d. Reporting a code for reimbursement

15. While the focus of inpatient data collection is on the principal diagnosis, the focus of outpatient data collection is on the:

    a. Reason for admission
    b. Activities of daily living
    c. Discharge diagnosis
    d. Reason for encounter

16. The inpatient data set incorporated into federal law and required for Medicare reporting is the:

    a. Ambulatory Care Data Set
    b. Uniform Hospital Discharge Data Set
    c. Minimum Data Set for Long-term Care
    d. Health Plan Employer Data and Information Set

17. Unstructured data may be preferred over structured data because:

    a. It does not require processing
    b. It provides greater detail
    c. Clinicians know how to enter it
    d. It is more complete

18. What document is a snapshot of a patient's status and includes everything from social issues to disease processes as well as critical paths and clinical pathways that focus on a specific disease process or pathway in a long-term care hospital (LTCH)?

    a. Face sheet
    b. Care plan
    c. Diagnosis plan
    d. Flow sheet

19. Which of the following personnel should be authorized, per hospital policy, to take a physician's verbal order for the administration of medication?

    a. Unit secretary working on the unit where the patient is located
    b. Nurse working on the unit where the patient is located
    c. Health information director
    d. Admissions registrars

20. Inadequate functions that make it impossible to detect when an entry was modified or borrowed from another source and misrepresented as an original entry by an authorized user is an example of a potential breach of:

    a. Authorship integrity
    b. Documentation integrity
    c. Auditing integrity
    d. Patient identification and demographic accuracy

21. Which health record format is arranged in chronological order with documentation from various sources intermingled?

    a. Electronic
    b. Source-oriented
    c. Problem-oriented
    d. Integrated

22. Which of the following represents data flow for a hospital inpatient admission?

    a. Registration > diagnostic and procedure codes assigned > services performed > charges recorded
    b. Registration > services performed > charges recorded > diagnostic and procedure codes assigned
    c. Services performed > charges recorded > registration > diagnostic and procedure codes assigned
    d. Diagnostic and procedure codes assigned > registration > services performed > charges recorded

23. Which of the following is the goal of quantitative analysis performed by health information management (HIM) professionals?

    a. Ensuring the record is legible
    b. Identifying deficiencies early so they can be corrected
    c. Verifying that health professionals are providing appropriate care
    d. Checking to ensure bills are correct

24. To complete a comprehensive assessment and collect information for the Minimum Data Set for Long-Term Care, the coordinator must use which of the following?

    a. Core measure
    b. Resident Assessment Instrument
    c. Precertification
    d. Record of transfer

25. Data content standards are used to:

    a. Share data in the same way the users interpret data
    b. Share data is a unique way
    c. Share data between disparate systems
    d. Modify data

26. A barrier to effective computer-assisted coding is the:

a. Resistance of physicians
b. Resistance of HIM professionals
c. Poor quality of documentation
d. Reduction of consistency without human coders

27. How do healthcare providers use the administrative data they collect?

a. For regulatory, operational, and financial purposes
b. For statistical data purposes
c. For electronic health record tracking purposes
d. For continuity of patient care purposes

28. Personal information about patients such as their names, ages, and addresses is considered what type of information?

a. Clinical
b. Administrative
c. Operational
d. Accreditation

29. Which of the following is ***not*** a benefit of electronic authentication executed at the completion of documentation within an application?

a. It saves time
b. Entries are stamped with time and date
c. It eliminates the possibility of documentation error
d. Entries are legible

30. A staghorn calculus of the left renal pelvis was treated earlier in the week by lithotripsy. The patient returns now for removal of the calculus via a percutaneous nephrostomy tube. What is the correct root operation?

a. Destruction
b. Extirpation
c. Fragmentation
d. Release

31. Changes and updates to ICD-10-CM are managed by the ICD-10-CM Coordination and Maintenance Committee, a federal committee cochaired by representatives from the NCHS and:

a. AMA
b. OIG
c. CMS
d. WHO

32. A computer software program that supports a coder in assigning correct codes is called a(n):

    a. Encoder
    b. Grouper
    c. Automated coder
    d. Decision support system

33. Mrs. Bolton is an angry patient who resents her physician "bossing her around." She refuses to take a portion of the medications the nurses bring to her pursuant to physician orders and is verbally abusive to the patient care assistants. Of the following options, the most appropriate way to document Mrs. Bolton's behavior in the patient health record is:

    a. Mean
    b. Noncompliant and hostile toward staff
    c. Belligerent and out of line
    d. A pain in the neck

34. Who is responsible for ensuring the quality of health record documentation?

    a. Board of directors
    b. Administrator
    c. Provider
    d. Health information management professional

35. Which of the following is an example of a 1:1 relationship?

    a. Patients to hospital admissions
    b. Patients to consulting physicians
    c. Patients to clinics
    d. Patients to hospital beds

36. The Joint Commission has published a list of abbreviations classified as "Do Not Use" for the purpose of:

    a. Assisting coders to read physician handwriting
    b. Preventing potential medication errors due to misinterpretation
    c. Making terminology consistent in preparation for electronic records
    d. Identifying physicians who are dispensing large quantities of drugs

37. According to the UHDDS definition, ethnicity should be recorded on a patient record as:

    a. Race of mother
    b. Race of father
    c. Spanish origin/Hispanic, non-Spanish origin/non-Hispanic, unknown
    d. Free-text descriptor as reported by patient

38. A patient with a diagnosis of ventral hernia is admitted to undergo a laparotomy with ventral hernia repair. The patient undergoes a laparotomy and develops bradycardia. The operative site is closed without the repair of the hernia. What is the correct code assignment?

I97.191	Other postprocedural cardiac functional disturbances following other surgery
K43.9	Ventral hernia without obstruction or gangrene
R00.1	Bradycardia, unspecified
Z53.09	Procedure and treatment not carried out because of other contraindication

Section	Body System	Root Operation	Body Part	Approach	Device	Qualifier
Medical and Surgical	Anatomical Regions, General	Repair	Abdominal Wall	Open	No Device	No Qualifier
0	W	Q	F	0	Z	Z

Section	Body System	Root Operation	Body Part	Approach	Device	Qualifier
Medical and Surgical	Anatomical Regions, General	Inspection	Peritoneal Cavity	Open	No Device	No Qualifier
0	W	J	G	0	Z	Z

a. K43.9, R00.1, Z53.09, 0WJG0ZZ
b. K43.9, I97.191, R00.1, 0WJG0ZZ
c. K43.9, 0WQF0ZZ
d. K43.9, Z53.09, 0WQF0ZZ

39. Which of the following is a component of the resident assessment instrument?

a. The resident's health record
b. A standard Minimum Data Set (MDS)
c. Preadmission Screening Assessment
d. Annual Resident Review

40. Each individual who has been authorized to document in the EHR uses a(n) ________ in the form of a code or password.

a. audit trail
b. digital signature
c. unique personal identifier
d. electronic signature

41. Which of the following is ***not*** an appropriate method for destroying paper-based health records?

a. Burning
b. Shredding
c. Pulverizing
d. Degaussing

42. Assign the correct CPT code for the following: A 63-year-old female had a temporal artery biopsy completed in the outpatient surgical center.

   a. 32405, Biopsy, lung or mediastinum, percutaneous needle
   b. 37609, Ligation or biopsy, temporal artery
   c. 20206, Biopsy, muscle, percutaneous needle
   d. 31629, Bronchoscopy, rigid or flexible, including fluoroscopic guidance when performed; with transbronchial needle aspiration biopsy(s), trachea, mainstem and/or lobar bronchus(i)

43. A diagnosis described as "possible," "probable," "likely," or "rule out" is reported as if present for which type of patient records?

   a. Outpatient
   b. Emergency room
   c. Physician office
   d. Inpatient

44. A patient returns during a 90-day postoperative period from a ventral hernia repair; the patient is now complaining of eye pain. What modifier would you use with the Evaluation and Management code?

   a. –79, Unrelated procedure or service by the same physician or other qualified health care professional during the postoperative period
   b. –25, Significant, separately identifiable evaluation and management service by the same physician or other qualified health care professional on the same day of the procedure or other service
   c. –59, Distinct procedural service
   d. –24, Unrelated evaluation and management service by the same physician or other qualified health care professional during a postoperative period

45. The legal health record for disclosure consists of:

   a. Any and all protected health information data collected or used by a healthcare entity when delivering care
   b. Only the protected health information requested by an attorney for a legal proceeding
   c. The data, documents, reports, and information that comprise the formal business records of any healthcare entity that are to be utilized during legal proceedings
   d. All of the data and information included in the HIPAA Designated Record Set

46. Which data set would be used to document an elective surgical procedure that does not require an overnight hospital stay?

   a. Uniform Hospital Discharge Data Set
   b. Data Elements for Emergency Department Systems
   c. Uniform Ambulatory Care Data Set
   d. Essential Medical Data Set

47. A patient was admitted to the hospital with symptoms of a stroke and secondary diagnoses of chronic obstructive pulmonary disease (COPD) and hypertension. The patient was subsequently discharged from the hospital with a principal diagnosis of cerebral vascular accident and secondary diagnoses of catheter-associated urinary tract infection, COPD, and hypertension. Which of the following diagnoses should ***not*** be reported as POA?

a. Catheter-associated urinary tract infection

b. Cerebral vascular accident

c. COPD

d. Hypertension

48. HIM professionals sometimes monitor the records of current inpatients as well as closed records after the patients have been discharged or transferred. What is this process called?

a. Qualitative record review

b. Legal record review

c. Quantitative record review

d. Ongoing record review

49. The purpose of the data dictionary is to ________ definitions and ensure consistency of use.

a. Identify

b. Standardize

c. Create

d. Organize

50. Which of the following is a graphical display of the relationships between tables in a database?

a. RDMS

b. SQL

c. ERD

d. SAS

51. It is important for a healthcare entity to have ________ addressing how to deal with corrections made to erroneous entries in health records.

a. Training sessions

b. Written procedures

c. Verbally communicated instructions

d. A supervisory committee

52. The process defined as signing multiple documents at one time without opening the documents, which falls short of federal and state authentication requirements and could place the healthcare entity at legal risk is called:

a. Autoauthentication

b. Manual authentication

c. Automated insertion

d. Proxy authentication

53. Assign the correct CPT code for the following: A 58-year-old male was seen in the outpatient surgical center for insertion of a self-contained inflatable penile prosthesis for impotence.

a. 54401, Insertion of penile prosthesis; inflatable (self-contained)

b. 54405, Insertion of multicomponent, inflatable penile prosthesis, including placement of pump, cylinders, and reservoir

c. 54440, Plastic operation of penis for injury

d. 54400, Insertion of penile prosthesis, noninflatable (semirigid)

54. Which of the following keywords precedes the listing of variables to be returned from an SQL query?

a. SELECT

b. SET

c. DATA

d. BY

55. An alteration of the health information by modification, correction, addition, or deletion is known as a(n):

a. Change

b. Amendment

c. Copy and paste

d. Deletion

56. A collection of data that is organized so its contents can be easily accessed, managed, and updated is called a:

a. Spreadsheet

b. Database

c. File

d. Data table

57. The process of providing proof of the authorship of health record documentation is called:

a. Identification

b. Standardization of data capture

c. Standardization of abbreviations

d. Authentication

58. Which of the following plans address how information can be documented in the health record during down time or a catastrophic event?

a. Disaster

b. E-discovery response

c. Business continuity

d. Emergency documentation

59. Which document is used in the long-term care setting that is ***not*** used in the acute-care setting?

a. Progress notes
b. Monthly summary
c. Physician consultations
d. Physician orders

60. Regardless of the healthcare setting, accreditation and regulatory standards require a separate healthcare record for each:

a. Family
b. Individual patient
c. Encounter with the facility
d. Day of treatment

61. A strategic plan that identifies applications, technology, and operational elements needed for the overall information technology program in a healthcare entity is a(n):

a. Implementation plan
b. Information technology plan
c. Migration path
d. Transition strategy

62. According to the Medicare Conditions of Participation, how long must health records be retained?

a. Two years
b. Five years
c. Ten years
d. Permanently

63. What is a legal document that is used to specify whether the patient would like to be kept on artificial life support if they become permanently unconscious or is otherwise dying and unable to speak for themselves?

a. Durable power of attorney
b. Living consent form
c. Informed consent
d. Advance directive

64. Which of the following is the appropriate method for destroying electronic data?

a. Burning
b. Shredding
c. Pulverizing
d. Degaussing

65. Records that are not completed by the physician within the time frame specified in the healthcare organization policies are called:

a. Default records
b. Delinquent records
c. Loose records
d. Suspended records

66. A patient born with a neural tube defect would be included in which type of registry?

a. Birth defects
b. Cancer
c. Diabetes
d. Trauma

67. Automated insertion of clinical data using templates or similar tools with predetermined components using uncontrolled and uncertain clinical relevance is an example of a potential breach of:

a. Patient identification and demographic accuracy
b. Authorship integrity
c. Documentation integrity
d. Auditing integrity

68. Which of the following is a business role with major responsibilities that include identifying the specific data needed to operate business processes, recording metadata, and identifying and enforcing quality standards?

a. Chief data officer
b. Data definition steward
c. Data production steward
d. Subject matter expert

69. Which of the following data management domains would be responsible for establishing standards for data retention and storage?

a. Data architecture management
b. Metadata management
c. Data life cycle management
d. Master data management

70. Records consisting of multiple electronic systems that do not communicate or are not logically architected for record management are called:

a. Electronic medical records
b. Electronic health records
c. Hybrid health records
d. Computerized health records

71. What is the primary advantage of using standardized data sets for collecting healthcare information?

a. Patients receive similar care in every facility

b. Data can be compared nationally

c. To ensure collection of complete information

d. To ensure quality information is documented

72. A pediatrician would report the fact that he or she administered the MMR vaccine to a toddler on a(n):

a. Diabetes registry

b. Cancer registry

c. Immunization registry

d. Trauma registry

73. Assign the correct CPT code for the following procedure: Revision of the pacemaker skin pocket.

a. 33223, Relocation of skin pocket for implantable defibrillator

b. 33210, Insertion or replacement of temporary transvenous single chamber cardiac electrode or pacemaker catheter (separate procedure)

c. 33212, Insertion of pacemaker pulse generator only; with existing single lead

d. 33222, Revision or relocation of skin pocket for pacemaker

74. The statement "All patients admitted with a diagnosis falling into ICD-10-CM code numbers S00 through T88" represents a possible case definition for what type of registry?

a. Birth defect registry

b. Cancer registry

c. Diabetes registry

d. Trauma registry

75. A database contains two tables: physicians and patients. If a physician may be linked to many patients and patients may only be related to one physician, what is the cardinality of the relationship between the two tables?

a. One-to-one

b. One-to-many

c. Many-to-many

d. One-to-two

76. Because a health record contains patient-specific data and information about a patient that has been documented by the professionals who provided care or services to that patient, it is considered:

a. Secondary data source

b. Aggregate data source

c. Primary data source

d. Reliable data source

77. The leadership and organizational structures, policies, procedures, technology, and controls that ensure that patient and other enterprise data and information sustain and extend the entity's mission and strategies, deliver value, comply with laws and regulations, minimize risk to all stakeholders, and advance the public good is called:

    a. Information asset management
    b. Information management
    c. Information governance
    d. Enterprise information management

78. Mary Smith, RHIA, has been charged with the responsibility of designing a data collection form to be used on admission of patients to the acute-care hospital in which she works. What is the first resource she should use?

    a. UHDDS
    b. UACDS
    c. MDS
    d. ORYX

79. What is the traditional paper format for a hospital patient care record?

    a. Integrated
    b. Practice-oriented
    c. Chronological
    d. Source-oriented

80. Secondary data sources provide information that is ________ available by looking at individual health records.

    a. not easily
    b. easily
    c. often
    d. never

81. When data is taken from the health record and entered into registries and databases, the data in the registries or databases is then considered a(n):

    a. Secondary data source
    b. Reliable data source
    c. Primary data source
    d. Unreliable data source

82. Which of the following are considered dimensions of data quality?

    a. Relevancy, granularity, timeliness, currency, accuracy, precision, and consistency
    b. Relevancy, granularity, timeliness, currency, atomic, precision, and consistency
    c. Relevancy, granularity, timeliness, concurrent, atomic, precision, and consistency
    d. Relevancy, granularity, equality, currency, precision, accuracy, and consistency

83. Appropriate documentation of health record destruction must be maintained permanently no matter how the process is carried out. This documentation usually takes the form of a:

a. Policy of destruction

b. Retention schedule

c. Regulation schedule

d. Certificate of destruction

84. What is a primary purpose for documenting and maintaining health records?

a. Effective communication among caregivers for continuity of care

b. Substantiate claims for reimbursement

c. Provide evidence for malpractice lawsuits

d. Contribute to medical science

85. Quality has several components, including appropriateness, technical excellence, ________, and acceptability.

a. Accuracy of diagnosis

b. Continuous improvement

c. Connectivity

d. Accessibility

86. The practices or methods that defend against charges questioning the integrity of the data and documents are called:

a. Authentication

b. Security

c. Accuracy

d. Nonrepudiation

87. Which of the following indexes would be used to compare the number and quality of treatments for patients who underwent the same operation with different surgeons?

a. Physician

b. Master patient

c. Procedure

d. Disease and operation

88. Review of disease indexes, pathology reports, and radiation therapy reports is part of which function in the cancer registry?

a. Case definition

b. Case finding

c. Follow-up

d. Reporting

89. The basic component of a(n) ________ is an object that contains both data and their relationships in a single structure.

  a. Object-oriented database
  b. Relational database
  c. Access database
  d. Structured database

90. What tool is used to sort data in a variety of ways to assist in the study of certain data elements?

  a. Registries
  b. Indexes
  c. Clinical trials
  d. Statistical reports

91. A critical early step in designing an EHR in which the characteristics of each data element are defined is to develop a(n):

  a. Accreditation manual
  b. Core content
  c. Continuity of care record
  d. Data dictionary

92. Dr. Jones dies while still in active medical practice. He leaves incomplete records at Medical Center Hospital. The best way for the HIM department to handle these incomplete records is to:

  a. Have the administrator of the hospital complete them
  b. Have the charge nurse on the respective nursing units complete them
  c. Ask the chief of staff to complete them
  d. File the incomplete records with a notation about the physician's death

93. The first deliverable from a legal health record (LHR) definition project is a:

  a. List of LHR stakeholders
  b. Document matrix of LHR components
  c. Letter of support from management
  d. Master source system matrix

94. In long-term care, the resident's care plan is based on data collected in the:

  a. UHDDS
  b. OASIS
  c. MDS
  d. HEDIS

95. The name of the government agency that has led the development of basic data sets for health records and computer databases is:

  a. The Centers for Medicare and Medicaid Services
  b. The National Committee on Vital and Health Statistics
  c. The American National Standards Institute
  d. The National Institute of Health

96. What term is used in reference to the systematic review of sample health records to determine whether documentation standards are being met?

a. Qualitative analysis
b. Legal record review
c. Utilization analysis
d. Ongoing record review

97. Which of the following is a concept designed to help standardize clinical content for sharing between providers?

a. Continuity of care record
b. Interoperability
c. Personal health record
d. SNOMED

98. Mary Smith delivers a stillborn infant at Medical Center Hospital. The appropriate method of documenting information about the infant is to:

a. Create a health record for the infant
b. File all infant information in the mother's record
c. Retain the infant's information in a separate administrative file
d. Not retain information about the infant in hospital records

99. A patient had a radical resection of soft tissue sarcoma of the left thigh. In ICD-10-PCS what would the root operation be for this procedure?

a. Excision
b. Repair
c. Resection
d. Destruction

100. A regular review of LHR policies and procedures to ensure a healthcare entity remains in compliance with legal requirements is generally called an LHR ________.

a. maintenance plan
b. management plan
c. attribute plan
d. strategic plan

101. Why is it important to extract individual patient information and enter it into a database?

a. To track the patient's health status
b. To review quality of healthcare services
c. To reveal patterns
d. To complete mandatory statistical reports

102. Where can you find guidelines for the retention and destruction of healthcare information?

a. Institute of Medicine
b. Municipal regulations
c. HIPAA
d. Accreditation standards

103. Sleeping patterns, head and chest measurements, feeding and elimination status, weight, and Apgar scores are recorded in which of the following records?

a. Obstetric
b. Newborn
c. Surgical
d. Emergency

104. This functionality can result in confusion from incessant repetition of irrelevant clinical data.

a. Change
b. Amendment
c. Copy and paste
d. Deletion

105. What is the first consideration in determining how long records must be retained?

a. The amount of space allocated for record filing
b. The number of records
c. The most stringent law or regulation in the state
d. The cost of filing space

Domain 2 *Information Protection: Access, Disclosure, Archival, Privacy, and Security*

106. To practice medicine, medical school students must pass a test before they can obtain a:

a. Degree
b. License
c. Residency
d. Specialty

107. Community Hospital wants to provide transcription services for transcription of office notes of the private patients of physicians. All of these physicians have medical staff privileges at the hospital. This will provide an essential service to the physicians as well as provide additional revenue for the hospital. In preparing to launch this service, the HIM director is asked whether a business associate agreement is necessary. Which of the following should the hospital HIM director advise to comply with HIPAA regulations?

a. Each physician practice should obtain a business associate agreement with the hospital.
b. The hospital should obtain a business associate agreement with each physician practice.
c. Because the physicians all have medical staff privileges, no business associate agreement is necessary.
d. Because the physicians are part of an Organized Health Care Arrangement (OHCA) with the hospital, no business associate agreement is necessary.

108. Which of the following is a mechanism that records and examines activity in information systems?

a. eSignature laws

b. Security audits

c. Minimum necessary rules

d. Access controls

109. A patient requests copies of her medical records in an electronic format. The hospital maintains a portion of the designated record set in a paper format and a portion of the designated record set in an electronic format. How should the hospital respond?

a. Provide the records in paper format only

b. Scan the paper documents so that all records can be sent electronically

c. Provide the patient with both paper and electronic copies of the record

d. Inform the patient that PHI cannot be sent electronically

110. The record custodian typically can testify about which of the following when a party in a legal proceeding is attempting to admit a health record as evidence?

a. The care provided to the patient

b. Identification of the record as the one subpoenaed

c. The qualifications of the treating physician

d. Identification of the standard of care used to treat the patient

111. If a healthcare provider is accused of breaching the privacy and confidentiality of a patient, what resource may a patient rely on to substantiate the provider's responsibility for keeping health information private?

a. Professional Code of Ethics

b. Federal Code of Fair Practice

c. Federal Code of Silence

d. State Code of Fair Practice

112. Which professional has the responsibility of determining when an individual or entity has the right to access healthcare information in a hospital setting?

a. Physicians

b. Nurses

c. Health information management professionals

d. Hospital administrators

113. Community Hospital is terminating its business associate relationship with a medical transcription company. The transcription company has no further need for any identifiable information that it may have obtained in the course of its business with the hospital. The CFO of the hospital believes that to be HIPAA compliant all that is necessary is for the termination to be in a formal letter signed by the CEO. In this case, how should the director of HIM advise the CFO?

a. Confirm that a formal letter of termination meets HIPAA requirements and no further action is required

b. Confirm that a formal letter of termination meets HIPAA requirements and no further action is required except that the termination notice needs to be retained for seven years

c. Confirm that a formal letter of termination is required and that the transcription company must provide the hospital with a certification that all PHI that it had in its possession has been destroyed or returned

d. Inform the CFO that business associate agreements cannot be terminated

114. Which process requires the verification of the educational qualifications, licensure status, and other experience of healthcare professionals who have applied for the privilege of practicing within a healthcare facility?

a. Deemed status

b. Judicial decision

c. Subpoena

d. Credentialing

115. Ensuring that data have been accessed or modified only by those authorized to do so is a function of:

a. Data integrity

b. Data quality

c. Data granularity

d. Logging functions

116. The federal physician self-referral statute is also known as the:

a. Sherman Anti-Trust Act

b. Deficit Reduction Act

c. False Claims Act

d. Stark Law

117. Community Hospital is planning implementation of various elements of the EHR in the next six months. Physicians have requested the ability to access the EHR from their offices and from home. What advice should the HIM director provide?

a. HIPAA regulations do not allow this type of access.

b. This access would be covered under the release of PHI for treatment purposes and poses no security or confidentiality threats.

c. Access can be permitted providing that appropriate safeguards are put in place to protect against threats to security.

d. Access cannot be permitted because the physicians would not be accessing information for treatment purposes.

118. The Medical Record Committee is reviewing the privacy policies for a large outpatient clinic. One of the members of the committee remarks that he feels that the clinic's practice of calling out a patient's full name in the waiting room is not in compliance with HIPAA regulations and that only the patient's first name should be used. Other committee members disagree with this assessment. What should the HIM director advise the committee?

a. HIPAA does not allow a patient's name to be announced in a waiting room.

b. There is no violation of HIPAA in announcing a patient's name, but the committee may want to consider implementing practices that might reduce this practice.

c. HIPAA allows only the use of the patient's first name.

d. HIPAA requires that patients be given numbers and that only the number be announced.

119. Which of the following is a kind of technology that focuses on data security?

a. Clinical decision support

b. Bitmapped data

c. Firewalls

d. Smart cards

120. Mr. Martin has asked his physician's office to review a copy of his PHI. His request must be responded to no later than ________ after the request was made.

a. 90 days

b. 60 days

c. 30 days

d. 6 weeks

121. A hospital currently includes the patient's social security number on the face sheet of the paper medical record and in the electronic version of the record. The hospital risk manager has identified this as a potential identity breach risk and wants the information removed. The physicians and others in the hospital are not cooperating, saying they need the information for identification and other purposes. Given this situation, what should the HIM director suggest?

a. Avoid displaying the number on any document, screen, or data collection field

b. Allow the information in both electronic and paper forms since a variety of people need this data

c. Require employees to sign confidentiality agreements if they have access to social security numbers

d. Contact legal counsel for advice

122. The Privacy Rule establishes that a patient has the right of access to inspect and obtain a copy of his or her PHI:

a. For as long as it is maintained

b. For six years

c. Forever

d. For 12 months

123. Under the HIPAA Security Rule, these types of safeguards have to do with protecting the environment:

a. Administrative
b. Physical
c. Security
d. Technical

124. Which of the following is ***not*** an identifier under the Privacy Rule?

a. Visa account 2773 985 0468
b. Vehicle license plate BZ LITYR
c. Age 75
d. Street address 265 Cherry Valley Road

125. One of the four general requirements a covered entity must adhere to in order to be in compliance with the HIPAA Security Rule is to:

a. Ensure the confidentiality, integrity, and addressability of ePHI
b. Ensure the confidentiality, integrity, and accuracy of ePHI
c. Ensure the confidentiality, integrity, and availability of ePHI
d. Ensure the confidentiality, integrity, and accountability of ePHI

126. In Medical Center Hospital's clinical information system, nurses may write nursing notes and may read all parts of the patient health record for patients on the unit in which they work. This type of authorized use is called:

a. Password limitation
b. Security clearance
c. Role-based access
d. User grouping

127. Which of the following controls external access to a network?

a. Access controls
b. Alarms
c. Encryption
d. Firewall

128. Which of the following must be reported to the medical examiner?

a. Burns
b. Accidental deaths
c. Causes of injury
d. Morbidity

129. HIPAA was designed to accomplish all of the following ***except***:

a. Designate HIM professionals as privacy officers
b. Establish a consistent set of privacy and security rules for healthcare information nationwide
c. Simplify the sharing of health information for legitimate purposes
d. Authorize that only the minimum necessary should be released upon proper authorization

130. Identifying appropriate users of specific information is a function of:

a. Access control
b. Nosology
c. Data modeling
d. Workflow modeling

131. A visitor sign-in sheet to a computer area is an example of what type of control?

a. Administrative
b. Audit
c. Facility access
d. Workstation

132. Which of the following is an administrative safeguard action?

a. Facility access control
b. Documentation retention guidelines
c. Maintenance record
d. Media reuse

133. Which of the following does ***not*** have to be included in a covered entity's notice of privacy practices?

a. Description with one example of disclosures made for treatment purposes
b. Description of all the other purposes for which a covered entity is permitted or required to disclose PHI without consent or authorization
c. Statement of individual's rights with respect to PHI and how the individual can exercise those rights
d. Patient's signature and e-mail address

134. What is the legal term used to define the protection of health information in a patient–provider relationship?

a. Access
b. Confidentiality
c. Privacy
d. Security

135. Mary Jones has been declared legally incompetent by the court. Mrs. Jones's sister has been appointed her legal guardian. Her sister requested a copy of Mrs. Jones's health records. Of the options listed here, what is the best course of action?

a. Comply with the sister's request but first request documentation from the sister that she is Mary Jones's legal guardian
b. Provide the information as requested by the sister
c. Require that Mary Jones authorize the release of her health information to the sister
d. Refer the sister to Mary Jones's doctor

136. Caitlin has been experiencing abdominal pain. Removal of her gallbladder was recommended. Who is responsible to obtain Caitlin's informed consent?

a. The anesthesiologist who will be administering general anesthesia
b. The surgical nurse who will assist during surgery
c. The physician who will be performing the surgery
d. The administrator in the surgery department

137. Health Insurance Portability and Accountability Act's Privacy Rule states that "________ used for the purposes of treatment, payment, or healthcare operations does not require patient authorization to allow providers access, use, or disclosure." However, only the ________ information needed to satisfy the specified purpose can be used or disclosed.

a. Demographic information, minimum necessary
b. Protected health information, minimum necessary
c. Protected health information, diagnostic
d. Demographic information, diagnostic

138. The HIM manager received notification that a user accessed the PHI of a patient with the same last name as the user. This is an example of a(n):

a. Encryption
b. Trigger flag
c. Transmission security
d. Redundancy

139. Which of the following is a direct command that requires an individual or a representative of a healthcare entity to appear in court or to present an object to the court?

a. Judicial decision
b. Subpoena
c. Credential
d. Regulation

140. Kay Denton wrote to Mercy Hospital requesting an amendment to her PHI. She states that her record incorrectly lists her weight at 180 lbs. instead of her actual 150 lbs., and amending it would look better on her record. The information is present on a copy of a history and physical that General Hospital sent to Mercy Hospital. Mercy Hospital may decline to grant her request based on which privacy rule provision?

a. Individuals do not have the right to make amendment requests.
b. The history and physical was not created by Mercy Hospital.
c. A history and physical is not part of the designated record set.
d. Mercy Hospital must grant her request.

141. Authorization management involves:

a. The process used to protect the reliability of a database
b. Limiting user access to a database
c. Allowing unlimited use of the database
d. Developing definitions for database elements

142. Per HITECH, an accounting of disclosures must include disclosures made during the previous:

a. 10 years

b. 6 years

c. 3 years

d. 1 year

143. In the case of behavioral healthcare information, a healthcare provider may disclose health information on a patient without the patient's authorization in which of the following situations?

a. Court order, duty to warn, and involuntary commitment proceedings

b. Duty to warn, release of psychotherapy notes, and court order

c. Involuntary commitment proceedings, court order, and substance abuse treatment records

d. Release of psychotherapy notes, substance abuse treatment records, and duty to warn

144. The age of majority in most states is:

a. 16 and older

b. 17 and older

c. 18 and older

d. 21 and older

145. City Hospital has implemented a procedure that allows inpatients to decide whether they want to be listed in the hospital's directory. The directory information includes the patient's name, location in the hospital, and general condition. If a patient elects to be in the directory, this information is used to inform callers who know the patient's name. Some patients have requested that they be listed in the directory but information is to be released to only a list of specific people the patient provides. A hospital committee is considering changing the policy to accommodate these types of patients. In this case, what type of advice should the HIM director provide?

a. Approve the requests because this is a patient right under HIPAA regulations

b. Deny these requests because screening of calls is difficult to manage and if information is given in error, this would be considered a violation of HIPAA

c. Develop two different types of directories—one directory for provision of all information and one directory for provision of information to selected friends and family of the patient

d. Deny these requests and seek approval from the Office of Civil Rights

146. A competent adult female has a diagnosis of ovarian cancer and while on the operating table suffers a stroke and is in a coma. Her son would like to access her health records from a clinic she recently visited for pain in her right arm. The patient is married and lives with her husband and two grown children. According to the Uniform Health Care Decisions Act (UHCDA), who is the logical person to request and sign an authorization to access the woman's health records from the clinic?

a. Adult child making request

b. Oldest adult child

c. Patient

d. Spouse

147. The baby of a mother who is 15 years old was recently discharged from the hospital. The mother is seeking access to the baby's health record. Who must sign the authorization for release of the baby's health record?

a. Both mother and father of the baby

b. Maternal grandfather of the baby

c. Maternal grandmother of the baby

d. Mother of the baby

148. The outpatient clinic of a large hospital is reviewing its patient sign-in procedures. The registration clerks say it is essential that they know if the patient has health insurance and the reason for the patient's visit. The clerks maintain that having this information on a sign-in sheet will make their jobs more efficient and reduce patient waiting time in the waiting room. What should the HIM director advise in this case?

a. To be HIPAA compliant, sign-in sheets should contain the minimal information necessary such as patient name.

b. Patient name, insurance status, and diagnoses are permitted by HIPAA.

c. Patient name, insurance status, and reason for visit would be considered incidental disclosures if another patient saw this information.

d. Any communication overheard by another patient is considered an incidental disclosure.

149. The Latin phrase meaning "let the master answer" that puts responsibility for negligent actions of employees on the employer is called:

a. *Res ipsa locquitor*

b. *Res judicata*

c. *Respondeat superior*

d. *Restitutio in integrum*

150. Employees in the hospital business office may have legitimate access to patient health information without patient authorization based on what HIPAA standard or principle?

a. Minimum necessary

b. Compound authorization

c. Accounting of disclosures

d. Preemption

151. Per the HITECH breach notification requirements, which of the following is the threshold in which the media and the Secretary of Health and Human Services should be notified of the breach?

a. more than 1,000 individuals affected

b. more than 500 individuals affected

c. more than 250 individuals affected

d. Any number of individuals affected requires notification

152. Dr. Williams is on the medical staff of Sutter Hospital, and he has asked to see the health record of his wife, who was recently hospitalized. Dr. Jones was the patient's physician. Of the options listed here, which is the best course of action?

a. Refer Dr. Williams to Dr. Jones and release the record if Dr. Jones agrees

b. Inform Dr. Williams that he cannot access his wife's health information unless she authorizes access through a written release of information

c. Request that Dr. Williams ask the hospital administrator for approval to access his wife's record

d. Inform Dr. Williams that he may review his wife's health record in the presence of the privacy officer

153. Which of the following are technologies and methodologies for rendering protected health information unusable, unreadable, or indecipherable to unauthorized individuals as a method to prevent a breach of PHI?

a. Encryption and destruction

b. Recovery and encryption

c. Destruction and redundancy

d. Interoperability and recovery

154. The hospital's public relations department in conjunction with the local high school is holding a job shadowing day. The purpose of this event is to allow high school seniors an opportunity to observe the various jobs in the hospital and to help the students with career planning. The public relations department asks for input on this event from the standpoint of HIPAA compliance. In this case, what should the HIM department advise?

a. Job shadowing is allowed by HIPAA under the provision of allowing students and trainees to practice.

b. Job shadowing should be limited to areas in which the likelihood of exposure to PHI is very limited, such as administrative areas.

c. Job shadowing is allowed by HIPAA under the provision of volunteers.

d. Job shadowing is specifically prohibited by HIPAA.

155. A hospital releases information to an insurance company with proper authorization by the patient. The insurance company forwards the information to a medical data clearinghouse. This process is referred to as:

a. Admissibility

b. Civil release

c. Privileging process

d. Redisclosure

156. When a patient revokes authorization for release of information after a healthcare entity has already released the information, the healthcare entity in this case:

a. May be prosecuted for invasion of privacy

b. Has become subject to civil action

c. Has violated the security regulations of HIPAA

d. Is protected by the Privacy Act

157. Generally, policies addressing the confidentiality of quality improvement (QI) committee data (minutes, actions, and so forth) state that this kind of data is:

  a. Protected from disclosure
  b. Subject to release with patient authorization
  c. Generally available to interested parties
  d. May not be reviewed or released to external reviewers such as the Joint Commission

158. An employer has contacted the HIM department and requested health information on one of his employees. Of the options listed here, what is the best course of action?

  a. Provide the information requested
  b. Refer the request to the attending physician
  c. Request the employee's written authorization for release of information
  d. Request the employer's written authorization for release of the employee's information

159. Under the HIPAA Privacy Rule, a hospital may disclose health information without authorization or subpoena in which of the following cases?

  a. The patient has been involved in a crime that may result in death.
  b. The patient has celebrity status and requires protection.
  c. The father of a 22-year-old is requesting the records.
  d. An attorney requests records.

160. Covered entities must retain documentation of their security policies for at least:

  a. Five years
  b. Five years from the date of origination
  c. Six years from the date when last in effect
  d. Six years from the date of the last incident

161. Under HIPAA, when is the patient's written authorization required to release his or her healthcare information?

  a. For purposes related to treatment
  b. For purposes related to payment
  c. For administrative healthcare operations
  d. For any purpose unrelated to treatment, payment, or healthcare operations

162. Notices of privacy practices must be available at the site where the individual is treated and:

  a. Must be posted next to the entrance
  b. Must be posted in a prominent place where it is reasonable to expect that patients will read them
  c. May be posted anywhere at the site
  d. Do not have to be posted at the site

163. According to the Privacy Rule, which of the following statements must be included in the notice of privacy practices?

a. A description (including at least one example) of the types of uses and disclosures the physician is permitted to make for marketing purposes.

b. A description of each of the other purposes for which the covered entity is permitted or required to use or disclose PHI without the individual's written consent or authorization.

c. A statement that other uses and disclosures will be made without the individual's written authorization and that the individual may not revoke such authorization.

d. A statement that all disclosures will be prohibited from future redisclosures.

164. Regarding an individual's right of access per HIPAA, a covered entity:

a. Must act on the request within 90 days

b. May extend its response by 60 days if it gives the reasons for the delay

c. May require individuals to make their requests in writing

d. Does not have limits regarding what it can charge individuals for copies of their health records

165. Central City Clinic has requested that Ghent Hospital send its hospital records from Susan Hall's most recent admission to the clinic for her follow-up appointment. Which of the following statements is true?

a. The Privacy Rule requires that Susan Hall complete a written authorization.

b. The hospital may send only discharge summary, history, and physical and operative report.

c. The Privacy Rule's minimum necessary requirement does not apply.

d. This "public interest and benefit" disclosure does not require the patient's authorization.

166. A federal confidentiality statute specifically addresses confidentiality of health information about ________ patients.

a. Developmentally disabled

b. Elderly

c. Drug and alcohol recovery

d. Cancer

167. The confidentiality of incident reports is generally protected in cases when the report is filed in:

a. The nursing notes

b. The patient's health record

c. The physician's progress notes

d. The hospital risk manager's office

168. Which one of the following has access to personally identifiable data without authorization or subpoena?

a. Law enforcement in a criminal case

b. The patient's attorney

c. Public health departments for disease reporting purposes

d. Workers' compensation for disability claim settlement

169. An original goal of HIPAA Administrative Simplification was to standardize:

a. Privacy notices given to patients

b. The electronic transmission of health data

c. Disclosure of information for treatment purposes

d. The definition of PHI

170. The privacy officer was conducting training for new employees and posed the following question to the trainees to help them understand the rule regarding protected health information (PHI): "Which of the following is an element that makes information 'PHI' under the HIPAA Privacy Rule?"

a. Identifies an attending physician

b. Specifies the insurance provider for the patient

c. Contained within a personnel file

d. Relates to one's health condition

171. To date, the HIM department has not charged for copies of records requested by the patient. However, the policy is currently under review for revision. One HIM committee member suggests using the copying fee established by the state. Another committee member thinks that HIPAA will not allow for copying fees. What input should the HIM director provide?

a. HIPAA does not allow charges for copying medical records.

b. Use the state formula because HIPAA allows hospitals to use the state formula.

c. Base charges on the cost of labor and supplies for copying and postage if copies are mailed.

d. Because HIPAA restricts charges to the cost of paper, charge only for the paper used for copying the records.

172. The technology, along with the policies and procedures for its use, that protects and controls access to ePHI are:

a. Administrative safeguards

b. Technical safeguards

c. Physical safeguards

d. Integrity controls

173. Which of the following is considered a two-factor authentication system?

a. User ID and password

b. User ID and voice scan

c. Password and swipe card

d. Password and PIN

174. Which of the following is a "public interest and benefit" exception to the authorization requirement?

a. Payment

b. PHI regarding victims of domestic violence

c. Information requested by a patient's attorney

d. Treatment

175. Which of the following statements is true in regard to training in protected health information (PHI) policies and procedures?

a. Every member of the covered entity's workforce must be trained.

b. Only individuals employed by the covered entity must be trained.

c. Training only needs to occur when there are material changes to the policies and procedures.

d. Documentation of training is not required.

176. Under the Privacy Rule, which of the following must be included in a patient accounting of disclosures?

a. State-mandated report of a sexually transmitted disease

b. Disclosure pursuant to a patient's signed authorization

c. Disclosure necessary to meet national security or intelligence requirements

d. Disclosure for payment purposes

177. Debbie, an HIM professional, was recently hired as the privacy officer at a large physician practice. She observes the following practices. Which is a violation of the HIPAA Privacy Rule?

a. Dr. Graham recommends a medication to a patient with asthma.

b. Dr. Herman gives a patient a pen with the name of a pharmaceutical company on it.

c. Dr. Martin recommends acupuncture to a patient.

d. Dr. Lawson gives names of asthma patients to a pharmaceutical company.

178. The Administrative Simplification portion of Title II of HIPAA addresses which of the following?

a. Creating standardized forms for release of information throughout the industry

b. Computer memory requirements for health plans maintaining patient health information

c. Security regulations for personal health records

d. Uniform standards for transactions and code sets

179. The HIPAA Privacy Rule permits charging patients for labor and supply costs associated with copying health records. Mercy Hospital is located in a state where state law allows charging patients a $100 search fee associated with locating records that have been requested. Which of the following statements is true when applied to this scenario?

a. State law will not be preempted in this situation.

b. The Privacy Rule will preempt state law in this situation.

c. The Privacy Rule never preempts existing state law.

d. The Privacy Rule always preempts existing state law.

180. ________ established the right of patients to access and amend their own health records.

a. HIPAA

b. Medicare

c. Medicaid

d. AHIMA

181. Lane Hospital has a contract with Ready-Clean, a local company, to come into the hospital to pick up all the facility's linens for off-site laundering. Ready-Clean is:

a. A business associate because Lane Hospital has a contract with it
b. Not a business associate because it is a local company
c. A business associate because its employees may see PHI
d. Not a business associate because it does not use or disclose individually identifiable health information

182. A healthcare entity that is governed by the HIPAA regulations is called a(n):

a. Authorized entity
b. Covered entity
c. Privacy entity
d. Regulated entity

183. Automated registration entries that generate erroneous patient identification—possibly leading to patient safety and quality of care issues, enabling fraudulent activity involving patient identity theft, or providing unjustified care for profit—is an example of a potential breach of:

a. Authorship integrity
b. Patient identification and demographic accuracy
c. Documentation integrity
d. Auditing integrity

184. A patient requests that disclosures made from her medical record be limited to specific clinical notes and reports. Given HIPAA requirements, how must the hospital respond?

a. The hospital must accept the request but does not have to agree to it.
b. The hospital must honor the request.
c. The hospital must guarantee that the request will be followed.
d. The hospital must agree to the request, providing that state or federal law does not prohibit it.

185. The privacy officer was conducting training for new employees and posed the following question to the trainees to help them understand the rule regarding breach notification: "If a breach occurs, which of the following must be provided to the individual whose PHI has been breached?"

a. The facility's notice of privacy practices
b. An authorization to release the individual's PHI
c. The types of unsecured PHI that were involved
d. A promise to never do it again

186. When should an e-discovery response team be formed?

a. When a healthcare entity can reasonably anticipate litigation
b. The team should be rebuilt yearly
c. Well in advance of any litigation
d. At least 30 days before the court date

187. Ted and Mary are the adoptive parents of Susan, a minor. What is the best way for them to obtain a copy of Susan's operative report?

a. Wait until Susan is 18

b. Present an authorization signed by the court that granted the adoption

c. Present an authorization signed by Susan's natural (birth) parents

d. Present an authorization that at least one of them (Ted or Mary) has signed

188. Per the Privacy Rule, which of the following requires authorization for research purposes?

a. Use of Mary's deidentified information about her myocardial infarction

b. Use of Mary's information about her asthma in a limited data set

c. Use of Mary's individually identifiable information related to her asthma treatments

d. Use of medical information about Jim, Mary's deceased husband

189. John Smith was seen in his primary care physician's office. When the provider attempted to call him with his laboratory results, he inadvertently called the incorrect John Smith and verbally provided him the lab result. Which of the following would apply to this situation in the context of breach notification?

a. The provider would be required to report the breach to the media.

b. No reporting is necessary because the laboratory results are not considered PHI and no breach can occur based on this fact.

c. Even though the results were discussed with the incorrect patient, no hard copy results were sent to the wrong person, so because the wrong John Smith could not keep the PHI, no reporting is necessary.

d. The provider would be required to report the breach to the Secretary of HHS.

190. Many states have mandatory reporting requirements for suspected abuse or mistreatment of the following categories of individuals:

a. Children, competent adults, and nursing home residents

b. Competent adults, residents of mental health facilities, and nursing home residents

c. Nursing home residents, the elderly, and residents of state mental health facilities

d. Residents of state mental health facilities, the elderly, and competent adults

191. What is the most common method for implementing entity authentication?

a. Personal identification number

b. Biometric identification systems

c. Token systems

d. Password systems

192. The health record of Kathy Smith, the plaintiff, has been subpoenaed for a deposition. The plaintiff's attorney wants to use the records as evidence to prove his client's case. In this situation, although the record constitutes hearsay, it may be used as evidence based on the:

a. Admissibility exception

b. Discovery exception

c. Direct evidence exception

d. Business records exception

193. Which landmark legal case established the responsibility of the hospital for the quality of care given by its physicians?

a. *Roe v. Wade*

b. *Darling v. Charleston Community Memorial Hospital*

c. *Brown v. Board of Education*

d. *Marbury v. Madison*

194. In all of the following situations PHI may be disclosed without providing the opportunity for an individual to object or to provide an authorization ***except***:

a. For disclosures for public health purposes as required by law

b. For disclosures to health oversight agencies as required by law

c. For reporting certain types of wounds or other physical injuries as required by law

d. For including the individual's name in the facility directory

195. A ________ helps a healthcare entity proactively ensure that the information they store and maintain is only being accessed in the normal course of business.

a. Contingency plan

b. Workflow analysis

c. Documentation audit

d. Security audit

196. Which of the following would be included in an accounting of disclosures?

a. Incidental to an otherwise permitted or required use disclosure

b. Disclosures to the individual about whom the information pertains

c. Disclosures made pursuant to an authorization

d. Patient information faxed to the bank

197. Which of the following is required in a risk analysis according to the Security Rule?

a. Determine the likelihood of threat occurrence and the potential impact

b. Focus on improved efficiency

c. Implement successful system migration and interoperability

d. Develop a sustainable business plan

198. An inherent weakness or absence of a safeguard that could be exploited by threat is a:

a. Security incident

b. Breach

c. Vulnerability

d. Threat

199. Which standard in the Security Rule provides guidance for covered entities to secure laptops and other small portable mobile technologies used within the healthcare facility?

a. Workstation security standard

b. Technical safeguard standard

c. Device and media controls standard

d. Facility access control standard

200. E-discovery rules were created in response to the tremendous volume of evidence maintained in electronic format that is pertinent to lawsuits and amended which legislation?

a. Federal Rules of Evidence
b. State Rules of Evidence
c. Federal Rules of Civil Procedure
d. State Rules of Civil Procedure

201. A subpoena *duces tecum* compels the recipient to:

a. Serve on a jury
b. Answer a complaint
c. Testify at a trial
d. Bring records to a legal proceeding

202. A valid subpoena *duces tecum* seeking health records does ***not*** have to:

a. Be signed by the plaintiff and defendant
b. Include the date, time, and place of the requested appearance
c. Include the case docket number
d. The name of the issuing attorney

203. Which of the following fundraising solicitations violates HIPAA?

a. One sent to cardiac patients only
b. One that includes opt-out instructions
c. One sent to all patients treated at a facility in the previous year
d. One preceded by a Notice of Privacy Practices that informed individuals about fundraising activity

204. Community Memorial Hospital is developing a new trauma center. The administrative team asks the director of HIM to ensure that hospital policies are in compliance with all regulations regarding acceptance and transfer of emergency patients. The legislation that the HIM director should review is the:

a. Prospective Payment Act
b. Health Insurance Portability and Accountability Act
c. Emergency Medical Treatment and Active Labor Act
d. Tax Equity and Fiscal Responsibility Act

205. According to the HIPAA Security Rule, how should a covered entity instruct a physician who needs a new smartphone when her current smartphone contains ePHI?

a. Keep her old smartphone
b. Turn in her old smartphone to have the memory wiped
c. Recycle the old smartphone by giving it to a charity
d. Do what she wants since IT is too busy with other projects

206. An employee accesses ePHI that does not relate to her job functions. What security mechanism should have been implemented to minimize this security breach?

a. Access controls
b. Audit controls
c. Contingency controls
d. Security incident controls

207. Which of the following is a best practice for protecting information that is text messaged?

a. Send a text message to more than one person
b. Enter a person's telephone number each time a text message is sent
c. Encrypt text messages during transmission
d. Presume that telephone numbers stored in memory remain valid

208. Training in PHI policies and procedures means that:

a. Every member of the covered entity's workforce must be trained
b. Only individuals employed by the covered entity must be trained
c. Training only needs to occur when there are material changes to the policies and procedures
d. Documentation of training is not required

209. The process that encodes textual material, converting it to scrambled data that must be decoded is a(n):

a. Audit trail
b. Encryption
c. Password
d. Physical safeguard

210. HITECH specifically includes all of the following as business associates ***except***:

a. Patient safety organizations
b. Health information exchanges
c. E-prescribing gateways
d. Facility housekeeping staff

211. When a competent adult refuses treatment, a court may be required to balance the individual's privacy interests against the:

a. Patient's level of pain
b. Physician's right to keep the patient alive
c. Government's interests in protecting human life
d. Provider's liability concerns

212. A nurse administrator who is not typically on call to cover staffing shortages gets called in over the weekend to staff the emergency department. She does not have access to enter notes since this is not a part of her typical role. In order to meet the intent of the HIPAA Security Rule, the hospital policy should include a:

a. Requirement for her to attend training before accessing ePHI

b. Provision for another nurse to share his or her password with the nurse administrator

c. Provision to allow her emergency access to the system

d. Restriction on her ability to access ePHI

213. Mrs. Guindon is requesting every piece of health information that exists about her from Garrett Hospital. The Garrett Hospital privacy officer must explain to her that, under HIPAA privacy regulations, she does not have the right to access her:

a. History and physical report

b. Operative report

c. Discharge summary

d. Psychotherapy notes

214. Which of the following presents the greatest risk of large-scale health information breaches?

a. Unlocked rooms

b. Computer monitors positioned toward high-traffic areas

c. Unattended computer workstations

d. Laptop theft

215. Which of the following statements is true with regard to responding to requests from individuals for access to their PHI?

a. A cost-based fee may be charged for retrieval of the PHI.

b. A cost-based fee may be charged for making a copy of the PHI.

c. No fees of any type may be charged.

d. A minimal fee may be charged for retrieval and copying of PHI.

216. According to HIPAA standards, designated individuals responsible for data security:

a. Must be identified by every covered entity

b. Are only required in large facilities

c. Are only required in hospitals

d. Are not required in small physician practices

217. Data security management involves defending or safeguarding:

a. Access to information

b. Data availability

c. Health record quality

d. System implementation

218. What type of safeguards comprise over half of all of the safeguards included in the Security Rule?

a. Physical safeguards
b. Technical safeguards
c. Administrative safeguards
d. Security safeguards

219. What is the most constant threat to health information integrity?

a. Natural threats
b. Environmental threats
c. Internal disaster
d. Humans

220. Which of the following statements about a firewall is ***false***?

a. It is a system or combination of systems that supports an access control policy between two networks.
b. The most common place to find a firewall is between the healthcare entity's internal network and the Internet.
c. Firewalls are effective for preventing all types of attacks on a healthcare system.
d. A firewall can limit internal users from accessing various portions of the Internet.

Domain 3 *Informatics, Analytics, and Data Use*

221. In order to effectively transmit healthcare data between a provider and a payer, both parties must adhere to which electronic data interchange standards?

a. DICOM
b. IEEE 1073
c. LOINC
d. X12N

222. The surgery department is evaluating its postoperative infection rate of 6 percent. The chief of surgery asks the quality improvement coordinator to find the postoperation infection rates of 10 similar hospitals in the same geographic region to see how the rates compare. This process is called:

a. Benchmarking
b. Critical pathway analysis
c. Internal comparisons
d. Universal precautions

223. This data collection tool is used when one needs to gather data on sample observations in order to detect patterns.

a. Check sheet
b. Ordinal data tool
c. Balance sheet
d. Nominal data tool

224. To ensure quality of data, the cancer committee reviews the abstracting done by the cancer registry personnel. This type of reliability check is called:

a. Precision
b. Recheck
c. Interrater
d. Construct

225. Which of the following are phases of the systems development life cycle (SDLC)?

a. Design, analysis, and alignment
b. Maintenance, implementation, and improvement
c. Analysis, design, and implementation
d. Analysis, alignment, and improvement

226. A researcher mined the Medicare Provider Analysis Review (MEDPAR) file. The analysis revealed trends in lengths of stay for rural hospitals. What type of investigation was the researcher conducting?

a. Content analysis
b. Effect size review
c. Psychometric assay
d. Secondary analysis

227. Which one of the following is an example of a clinical information system?

a. Laboratory information system
b. Human resource management system
c. Patient registration system
d. Staff management system

228. The following graph of data security breaches shows a range of breaches from year one (YR-1) to year seven (YR-7). In year four (YR-4), a law came into effect for the mandatory reporting of security breaches. Given this information, which of the following is the best interpretation of the graph?

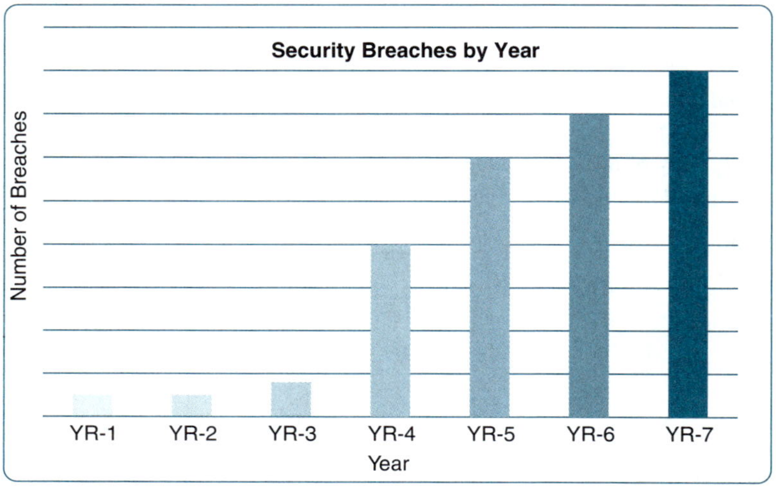

a. Between YR-2 and YR-3, there were very few data security breaches.
b. Security breaches were less prevalent from YR-4 to YR-7.
c. The volume of security breaches cannot be adequately estimated prior to YR-4.
d. In YR-4 there were more security breaches than YR-7.

229. Which of the following terms is defined as the proportion of people in a population who have a particular disease at a specific point in time or over a specified period of time?

a. Prevalence
b. Incidence
c. Frequency
d. Distribution

230. A director of a health information services department plans to do a research project on motivation that involves rewarding some employees for achieving specified goals. A control group will not be rewarded for achieving the same goals. Which entity will need to approve this study?

a. Institutional Review Board
b. Administrative team
c. Accreditation organization
d. Medical staff

231. A research instrument that is used to gather data and information from respondents in a uniform manner through the administration of a predefined and structured set of questions and possible responses is called a(n):

a. Survey
b. Interview
c. Process measure
d. Affinity diagram

232. This type of chart is used to focus attention on any variation in a process and helps the team to determine whether that variation is normal or a result of special circumstances.

a. Pareto chart

b. Pie chart

c. Control chart

d. Line chart

233. What is the average of the sum of the relative weights of all patients treated during a specified time period?

a. Case-mix index

b. Outlier pool

c. Share

d. Mean qualifier

234. Standardized sets of valid, reliable, and evidence-based measures implemented by the Joint Commission are called:

a. Sentinel events

b. Indicator monitoring systems

c. Core (performance) measures

d. Technical reporting requirements

235. The process of preventing the spread of communicable diseases in compliance with applicable legal requirements is performed in this quality management function.

a. Infection control

b. Clinical quality assessment

c. Utilization management

d. Risk management

236. Which of the following best describes the intent of strategic information systems planning?

a. Provide the potential for growth and expansion

b. Ensure that all information technology initiatives are integrated and aligned with the healthcare entity's overall strategy

c. Assess community or market needs and resources

d. Ensure ongoing accreditation

237. The HIM director is performing a staffing analysis to determine the number of employees needed to prep, scan, index, and carry out quality control on scanned medical records. Given a turnaround time of 24 hours and an average number of 48,000 images to be captured and considering the benchmarks listed here, what is the least number of employees the department needs, with each employee working an eight-hour shift?

Benchmarks for Document Scanning Processes

Function	Expectations per Worked Hour
Prepping	340–500 images
Scanning	1,200–2,400 images
Quality Control	1,600–2,000 images
Indexing	600–800 images

a. 25 employees
b. 36 employees
c. 36.1 employees
d. 37 employees

238. Which of the following is the statistic that would be used to explore the relationship between length of stay and patient age?

a. Mean
b. Correlation
c. Predictive modeling
d. Variance

239. A ________ is a range of values, such that the probability of that range covering the true value of a parameter is a set probability or confidence.

a. Confidence interval
b. Hypothesis
c. Proportion
d. Median

240. What is the term for health records maintained by patients or their families?

a. Electronic health records
b. Mixed-media records
c. Personal health records
d. Longitudinal health records

241. The distribution in this curve is:

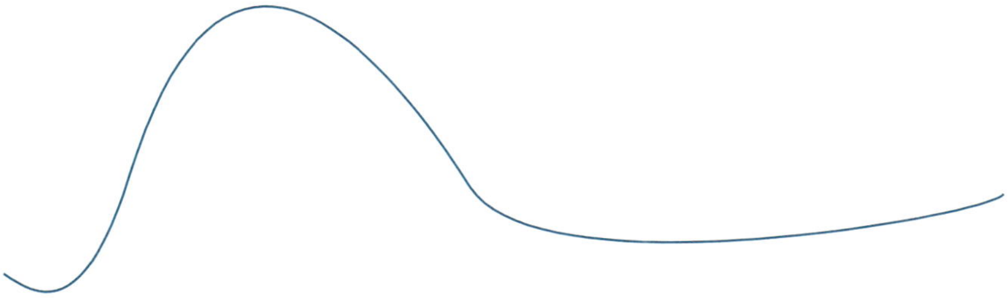

a. Normal

b. Bimodal

c. Skewed left

d. Skewed right

242. The following table shows the LOS for a sample of 11 discharged patients. Using the data listed, calculate the range.

Patient	Length of Stay
1	1
2	3
3	5
4	3
5	2
6	29
7	3
8	4
9	2
10	1
11	2

a. 29

b. 1

c. 5

d. 28

243. Which application uses statistical techniques to determine the likelihood of certain events occurring together?

a. Predictive modeling

b. Standard deviation

c. T-test

d. Serial numbering

244. This statistical inference measures both the strength of a relationship between two variables and the functional relationship between them.

a. Correlation

b. T-test

c. Simple linear regression

d. Standard deviation

245. The generic formula for calculating rate of occurrence is used to calculate hospital-acquired infections in an intensive care unit in a given month. If the number of hospital-acquired infections is the numerator, the denominator would be the:

a. Number of patients who died of infection

b. Number of deaths in the ICU

c. Number of discharges (including deaths) of ICU patients

d. Total number of hospital discharges

246. A hospital allows the use of the copy functionality in its EHR system for documentation purposes. The hospital has established explicit policies that define when the copy function may be used. Which of the following would be the best approach for conducting a retrospective analysis to determine if hospital copy policies are being followed?

a. Randomly audit EHR documentation for patients readmitted within 30 days.

b. Survey practitioners to determine if they are following hospital policy.

c. Institute an in-service program for all hospital personnel.

d. Observe the documentation practices of all clinical personnel.

247. This type of data display tool is used to illustrate frequency distributions of continuous variables, such as age or length of stay (LOS).

a. Bar graph

b. Histogram

c. Pie chart

d. Scatter diagram

248. How long should the master patient index be maintained?

a. For at least 5 years

b. For at least 10 years

c. For at least 25 years

d. Permanently

249. A technique that describes an interaction between a user and a system is called a(n):

a. Use case analysis

b. RHIO

c. Test case

d. Use description

250. The patient accounting department at Wildcat Hospital is concerned because last night's bill drop contained half the usual number of inpatient cases. Which of the following reports will be most useful in determining the reason for the low volume of bills?

a. Accounts receivable aging report
b. Discharged, no final bill report
c. Case-mix index report
d. Discharge summary report

251. Suppose that you are purchasing shelving units. The department has planned for units that are 5 shelves high, and each shelf is to be 36 inches wide and have 33 inches of actual filing space. From a sampling of records in the current files, you have determined that the average thickness of each record is 2 inches. You are planning to store 10 years' worth of records, and the average discharge rate is 2,000 per year. How many shelving units do you need to purchase?

a. 165
b. 180
c. 242
d. 243

252. In the following figure there is:

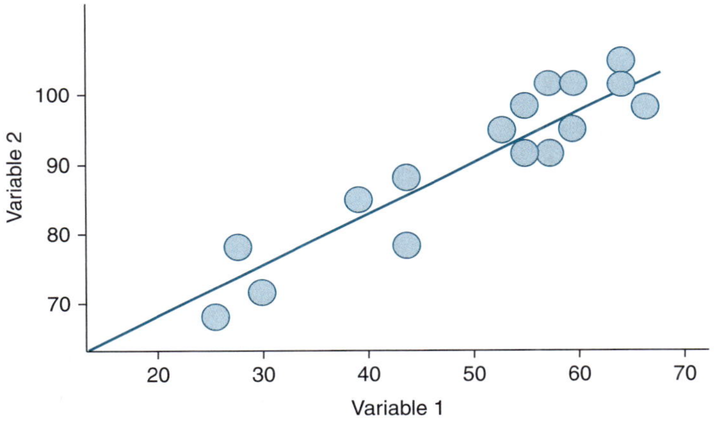

a. No correlation between the variables
b. A negative relationship between the variables
c. A weak negative correlation between the variables
d. A positive relationship between the variables

253. A measure of variability that describes the deviation from the mean of a frequency distribution in the original units of measurement is called the:

a. Mean
b. Mode
c. Standard deviation
d. Standard variance

254. A current key function in the health information field whereby data is turned into useful information is:

a. Data mining

b. Decision analysis

c. Clinical decision support

d. Data analytics

255. What term is used for a centralized database that captures, sorts, and processes patient data and then sends it back to the user?

a. Clinical data repository

b. Data exchange standard

c. Central processor

d. Digital system

256. Dr. Jones comes into the HIM department and requests that the HIM director pull all of his records from the previous year in which the principal diagnosis of myocardial infarction was indicated. Where would the HIM director begin to pull these records?

a. Disease index

b. Master patient index

c. Operative index

d. Physician index

257. In analyzing the reason for changes in a hospital's Medicare case-mix index over time, the analyst should start with which of the following levels of detail?

a. Account level

b. MS-DRG level

c. MDC level

d. MS-DRG triples, pairs, and singles

258. A healthcare entity remains committed to purchasing a vendor's product, which the entity finds solid in its financial and administrative applications but weaker in clinical applications. What is the term for this strategy?

a. Bridge

b. Best-of-fit

c. Best-of-breed

d. Legacy

259. In January, Community Hospital had 57 discharges from its medicine unit. Four patients developed urinary tract infections while in the hospital. What is the hospital-acquired infection rate for the medicine unit for January?

a. 0.07 %

b. 2.17 %

c. 7 %

d. 217 %

260. The HIM director is on the design team for the CPOE system. During a user interface design session, a sample of the electronic system is demonstrated. Two of the physicians are concerned about the overuse of alerts. What problem could the alert feature pose in the new system?

a. Unnecessary alerts can lead to clinicians ignoring other important alerts.

b. Alerts make order entry difficult.

c. Physicians do not like to be reminded how to treat patients.

d. The Joint Commission discourages an alert system.

261. In which phase of the systems development life cycle does initial training on a new information system generally occur?

a. Analysis

b. Design

c. Implementation

d. Maintenance and evaluation

262. Identifying user information needs is part of which phase of the systems development life cycle?

a. Analysis

b. Design

c. Implementation

d. Evaluation

263. The ________ is a standardized assessment of consumer perspectives regarding healthcare access and quality in hospitals.

a. HCAHPS

b. CG-CAHPS

c. AHRQ-CAHPS

d. ONC-CAHPS

264. The capture of secondary diagnoses that increase the incidence of CCs and MCCs at final coding may have an impact on:

a. Query rate

b. Principal diagnosis

c. Case-mix index

d. Record review rate

265. In which type of health information exchange architectural model does the entity operate much like an application service provider (ASP) or bank vault?

a. Consolidated

b. Federated—consistent databases

c. Federated—inconsistent databases

d. Switch

266. Community Memorial Hospital discharged nine patients on April 1. The length of stay for each patient is shown in the following table. What is the median length of stay for this group of patients?

Patient	Length of Stay, in Days
A	1
B	5
C	3
D	3
E	8
F	8
G	8
H	9
I	9

a. 5 days
b. 6 days
c. 8 days
d. 9 days

267. Last year, 73,249 people died from diabetes mellitus in the United States. The total number of deaths from all causes was 2,443,387, and the total population was 288,356,713. Calculate the proportionate mortality ratio for diabetes mellitus.

a. 0.003
b. 10.94
c. 0.09
d. 3.0

268. Which index, often considered the most important resource in a healthcare facility, is a database of patients within the facility or associated group of facilities?

a. Facility-specific index
b. Disease index
c. Master patient index
d. Operation index

269. Which of the following basic services provided by a health information exchange (HIE) entity matches identifying information to an individual?

a. Consent management
b. Person identification
c. Record locator
d. Identity management

270. Dictated and transcribed reports and notes written by the physicians and other practitioners are examples of:

a. Standardized clinical information

b. Codified data

c. Aggregate data

d. Unstructured clinical information

271. Allowing different health information systems to work together within and across organizational boundaries is referred to as:

a. Telehealth

b. Interoperability

c. Informatics

d. Interfaces

272. The purpose of Regional Extension Centers is to:

a. Implement meaningful use

b. Support providers in adopting EHR and with technical assistance

c. Develop standards for HI systems

d. Provide funding for expanding the adoption of HI technology

273. One strategy for acquiring EHR components from various vendors and interfacing them is:

a. Best-of-breed

b. Best-of-fit

c. Dual core

d. Integration

274. This EHR implementation strategy stops its paper processing immediately after the go-live of the system.

a. Phased roll-out

b. Big bang roll-out

c. Pilot

d. Straight turnover

275. Protocols that support communication between applications are often referred to as:

a. Application program

b. Interface code

c. Messaging standards

d. Source code

276. Which of the following basic services provided by an HIE entity identifies participating users and systems?

a. Identity management

b. Person identification

c. Registry and directory

d. Secure data transport

277. Which of the following is true of the median?

a. It is a measure of variability.
b. It is difficult to calculate.
c. It is based on the whole distribution.
d. It is sensitive to extreme values.

278. Mary Smith, RHIA, director of HIM at Central Hospital is in the process of training staff and employees on the move from a paper record to an electronic record. As she continues this transition, what health record format would most likely be used?

a. Hybrid records
b. Integrated records
c. Problem-oriented records
d. Clinical decision records

279. An EKG tracing is an example of ________ data.

a. Structured
b. Bit-mapped
c. Free text
d. Vector graphic

280. Data mining is a process that involves which of the following?

a. Using reports to measure outcomes
b. Using sophisticated computer technology to sort through an entity's data to identify unusual patterns
c. Producing summary reports for management to run the daily activities of the healthcare entity
d. Producing detailed reports to track productivity

281. Providers who do not implement an EHR will eventually be penalized through:

a. Reduction in Medicare payments
b. Reduction in amount of reimbursement from private insurance programs
c. Increased administrative costs to process claims
d. Restrictions from providing some patient care services

282. A secure method of communication between the healthcare provider and the patient is:

a. Personal health record
b. E-mail
c. Patient portal
d. Online health information

283. This EHR turnover strategy continues with its paper processing until the EHR works as planned.

a. Parallel processing
b. Phased roll-out
c. Pilot
d. Straight turnover

284. A key element in effective systems implementation is:

a. Contract negotiation
b. User training
c. System evaluation
d. RFP analysis

285. Which type of architecture has one powerful central computer that performs all processing and storage functions while sending and receiving data to or from various terminals and printers?

a. Client or server
b. Mainframe
c. Super computer
d. Web-based

286. The term used to describe breaking data elements into the level of detail needed to retrieve the data is:

a. Normalization
b. Data definitions
c. Primary key
d. A database management system

287. What is the most important factor in determining the best storage method for health records?

a. Ensuring that the records are readily accessible and secure
b. Ensuring that the records are factual and informational
c. Ensuring that the records are both electronic and paper based
d. Ensuring that the records are personal and private

288. A protocol to pass data from the system of one vendor to the information system of another vendor is called:

a. OLAP
b. Integration
c. TCP/IP
d. Interface

289. What technology creates images of handwritten and printed documents that are then stored in health record databases as electronic files?

a. Clinical data repository
b. Data exchange standards
c. Central processor
d. Digital scanner

290. Fifty percent of patients treated at our facilities have Medicare as their primary payer. This is an example of what type of information?

a. Patient-specific

b. Expert knowledge

c. Comparative

d. Aggregate

291. The probability of making a Type I error based on a particular set of data is called the ________.

a. Sampling value

b. Hypothesis test

c. A-probability

d. P-value

292. What must be in place to enhance the retrieval process for scanned documents?

a. Electronic signature

b. Indexing system

c. RFID device

d. Table of contents

293. All computers on this type of network receive the same message at the same time, but only one computer at a time can transfer information; and if one segment of the network goes down, the entire network is affected.

a. Star topology

b. Ring topology

c. Bus topology

d. Logical topology

294. What is an advantage of the unit numbering system?

a. All records for a specific patient, both inpatient and outpatient, are kept together.

b. The charts have to be split into volumes for filing.

c. The hospital can accommodate a large outpatient clinic with many return visits.

d. Joint Commission approval is automatic because all parts of the record are filed together.

295. When describing the typical length of stay for patients admitted for congestive heart failure, which is the most appropriate measure of central tendency when there are a number of long stay outliers?

a. Minimum

b. Mean

c. Median

d. Mode

296. The most common architecture used in EHRs in hospitals today is:

a. Client or server

b. Mainframe

c. Network computers

d. Web-based

297. In addition to bar codes on health record documents, what other forms of recognition characteristics enhance the accuracy of form indexing features?

a. Access controls

b. COLD

c. OCR

d. Workflow

298. All of the following are a kind of technology that focuses on data security ***except*** ________.

a. Encryption

b. Biometrics

c. Firewalls

d. Telemedicine

299. Which of the following statements is true of structured query language (SQL)?

a. It is both a data manipulation and data back-up mechanism.

b. It defines data elements and manipulates and controls data.

c. It is the computer language associated with document imaging.

d. Users are not able to query a relational database.

300. An evaluation of the benefits that have accrued from the EHR investment that is performed at specific milestones in the life of the project and used to help in future systems planning, designing, and implementing is called a:

a. Benefits realization study

b. Goal-setting exercise

c. Cost–benefit feasibility study

d. Productivity improvement study

301. The process of recouping lost data or reconciling conflicting data after a system failure is called:

a. Data backup

b. Data mapping

c. Data recovery

d. Data warehouse

302. Which of the following is an example of an e-health application?

a. Bedside nursing care

b. Appointment scheduling

c. Direct patient care

d. Emergency care records

303. In which record numbering system is the patient assigned a health record number on the first visit that is kept for all subsequent visits?

a. Unit numbering

b. Index unit numbering

c. Serial-unit numbering

d. Serial numbering

304. A single point of personalized web access through which to find and deliver information, applications, and services is called a(n):

a. Keyhole
b. Entry way
c. WWW
d. Portal

305. The process of integrating healthcare facility systems requires the creation of:

a. Data warehouses
b. E-health initiatives
c. Enterprise master patient indexes
d. Electronic data interchange

306. In this type of network configuration, individual computers are connected through a central hub that serves as a traffic cop for the data.

a. Star topology
b. Ring topology
c. Bus topology
d. Logical topology

307. For an EHR to provide robust clinical decision support, what critical element must be present?

a. Structured data
b. Internet connection
c. Physician portal
d. Standard vocabulary

308. The computer abstracting system in a facility has an edit that does not allow coders to assign obstetrical codes to male patients. This edit is called a(n):

a. Preventive control
b. Feedback control
c. Performance measure
d. Audit trail

309. Community Hospital just added a new system that changed the way data move throughout the facility. Which of the following would need to be updated to reflect this change?

a. Data dictionary
b. Entity relationship diagram
c. Data flow diagram
d. Semantic object model

310. The benefits patients experience when using a patient portal include all of the following ***except*** being able to:

a. Edit their medical record information

b. View lab results

c. Update demographics

d. Send messages to their providers

311. Which of the following is ***not*** a statistical technique used to create a model to assess the probability that current Medicare claims are fraudulent?

a. Logistic regression

b. Cluster analysis

c. Decision trees

d. Database warehousing

312. In order for health information exchange (HIE) participants to search for health records on each of the other systems using patient indexing and identification software, the systems must be linked by a(n):

a. Primary key interface (PKI)

b. Application programming interface (API)

c. Continuity of care record (CCR)

d. Record locator service (RLS)

313. In this EHR implementation strategy, virtually every nursing unit, department, clinic, or other organizational unit goes live at the same time with a given component of the EHR.

a. Phased roll-out

b. Big bang roll-out

c. Pilot

d. Straight turnover

314. Which numerical filing system results in an even distribution of records and ensures activity throughout the filing area?

a. Serial-unit filing system

b. Serial filing system

c. Unit filing system

d. Terminal-digit filing system

315. Which of the following is an organization that develops standards related to the interoperability of health information technology?

a. National Health Information Network

b. National Committee on Vital and Health Statistics

c. Health Level 7

d. EHR Collaborative

316. A network made accessible to trusted individuals outside of the facility is called a(n):

a. Extranet
b. Intranet
c. VPN
d. LAN

317. The Joint Commission requirement regarding delinquent records is that the number of delinquent records in a facility cannot exceed:

a. 50 per week
b. 2,000 per year
c. 50 percent of the average number of discharges
d. 25 percent of yearly admissions

318. Which of the following are used by an organization or enterprise to determine the probability of a duplicate data element to identify potential duplicate MPI entries?

a. Patient interviews
b. Addendums
c. Algorithms
d. Physician queries

319. All of the following are necessary to maintain an accurate MPI in an EHR environment ***except***:

a. Standardizing registration procedures
b. Training all registration staff
c. Identifying registration entry points
d. Assigning registry accession numbers

320. Consumer informatics is focused on ________

a. Consumer activation
b. Information structures and processes
c. Personalized medicine
d. Engagement

321. If a health plan analyst wanted to determine if the readmission rates for two hospitals were statistically different, what is the null hypothesis?

a. The readmission rates are not equal.
b. The readmission rates are equal.
c. The readmission rate for one hospital is larger than the other.
d. The readmission rate for one hospital is smaller than the other.

322. Which of the following lists represents recommended core data elements for the master patient index?

a. Date of birth, revenue code, accession number, and address
b. Name, address, revenue code, and accession number
c. Name, gender, address, and date of birth
d. Gender, address, accession number, and charge code

323. Laboratory data are successfully transmitted back and forth from Community Hospital to three local physician clinics. This successful transmission is dependent on which of the following standards?

a. X12N

b. LOINC

c. RxNorm

d. DICOM

324. Which of the following ensures that procedures are in place to handle an emergency response in the event of an untoward event such as a power outage?

a. An audit control

b. A contingency plan

c. Employee training

d. Password protection

325. In which of the following does an analyst perform exploratory data analysis to determine trends and identify patterns in the data set?

a. Data quality

b. Data mining

c. Record analysis

d. Inferential statistics

326. A radiology department is planning to develop a remote clinic and plans to transmit images for diagnostic purposes. The most important set of standards to implement in order to transmit images is:

a. X12N

b. LOINC

c. IEEE 1073

d. DICOM

327. An analyst wishes to test the hypothesis that the wait time in the emergency department is longer on weekends than weekdays. What is the alternative hypothesis?

a. The average wait time is shorter on weekends.

b. The average wait time is longer on weekends.

c. The average wait time is different on weekends and weekdays.

d. The average wait time is the same on weekends and weekdays.

328. Which graph is the best choice to use when exploring the relationship between length of stay and charge for a set of patients?

a. Line graph

b. Bar chart

c. Pie chart

d. Scatter diagram

329. Which of the following is the goal of an MPI ongoing maintenance program?

a. To maintain low creation rates for duplicates, overlaps, and overlays
b. To maintain the readmission rate for the facility
c. To carry out treatment, payment, and operations
d. To ensure appropriate state regulations of insurance and health plans

330. Which model for health information exchange stores patient records in a single database built to allow queries into the system?

a. Federated
b. Hybrid
c. Centralized
d. Decentralized

331. An analyst wishes to use the CMI for a set of MS-DRGs to determine if a documentation improvement program is having an impact. Use the MS-DRG volumes and weights in the table below to calculate the CMI for the three MS-DRGs.

MS-DRG	Description	Weight	Volume
034	CAROTID ARTERY STENT PROCEDURE W MCC	3.6918	100
035	CAROTID ARTERY STENT PROCEDURE W CC	2.1965	52
036	CAROTID ARTERY STENT PROCEDURE W/O CC/MCC	1.6610	36

a. 2.3234
b. 2.8893
c. 2.5164
d. 3.6918

Domain 4 *Revenue Management*

332. Which of the following statements about new technology items included on the charge description master (CDM) is ***false***?

a. The CDM maintenance committee should review new technology items for FDA approval.
b. The CDM maintenance committee should review new technology items for OPPS pass-through assignment.
c. The CDM maintenance committee should have a professional coder review code assignments even if codes are suggested by the manufacturer.
d. The codes for new technology should not be included in the CDM until coverage has been determined.

333. Patient accounting is reporting an increase in national coverage decisions (NCDs), and local coverage determinations (LCDs) failed edits in observation accounts. Which of the following departments will be tasked to resolve this issue?

a. Utilization management
b. Patient access
c. Health information management
d. Patient accounts

334. The discharged, not final billed report (also known as discharged, no final bill or accounts not selected for billing or DNFB) includes what types of accounts?

a. Accounts that have been discharged and have not been billed for a variety of reasons

b. Only discharged inpatient accounts awaiting generation of the bill

c. Only uncoded patient records

d. Accounts that are within the system hold days and not eligible to be billed

335. Patient accounts has submitted a report to the revenue cycle team detailing $100,000 of outpatient accounts that are failing NCD edits. All attempts to clear the edits have failed. There are no ABNs on file for these accounts. Based only on this information, the revenue cycle team should:

a. Bill the patients for these accounts

b. Contact the patients to obtain an ABN

c. Write off the accounts to contractual allowances

d. Write off the failed charges to bad debt and bill Medicare for the clean charges

336. Under RBRVS, which elements are used to calculate a Medicare payment?

a. Work value and extent of the physical exam

b. Malpractice expenses and detail of the patient history

c. Work value and practice expenses

d. Practice expenses and review of systems

337. In reviewing a patient chart, the coder finds that the patient's chest x-ray is suggestive of chronic obstructive pulmonary disease (COPD). The attending physician mentions the x-ray finding in one progress note, but no medication, treatment, or further evaluation is provided. Which of the following actions should the coder take in this case?

a. Query the attending physician and ask him to validate a diagnosis based on the chest x-ray results

b. Code COPD because the documentation substantiates it

c. Query the radiologist to determine whether the patient has COPD

d. Assign a code from the abnormal findings to reflect the condition

338. The following are the most common reasons for claim denials ***except*** ________.

a. Billing noncovered services

b. Lack of medical necessity

c. Beneficiary not covered

d. Coverage not in effect for date of service

339. Using the information provided, if the physician is a non-PAR who accepts assignment, how much can he or she expect to be reimbursed by Medicare?

> Physician's normal charge = $340
> Medicare Fee Schedule = $300
> Patient has met his deductible

a. $228

b. $240

c. $285

d. $300

340. An outcome of coding audit reviews may be any of the following ***except***:

a. Coding documentation issues that prevent the coders from performing comprehensive coding are identified

b. Redundant codes on the claims are identified

c. Cases where excellent penmanship created challenges for the coders are identified

d. Areas where coding could be improved if a physician was queried are identified

341. Long-term care hospitals must meet state requirements for ________ and have an agreement with ________ in order to receive payments.

a. Acute care hospitals, Medicare

b. Medicare, acute care hospitals

c. Fiscal intermediaries, Medicare

d. Medicare, fiscal intermediaries

342. The universal protocol requires a "time-out" prior to the start of any surgical or invasive procedure to conduct a verification of:

a. Patient and procedure

b. Patient, procedure, and site

c. Surgeon and site

d. Surgeon, patient, and site

Use the following figure for questions 343 and 344:

343. From the figure, determine whether the plan covers Gill F. White, Jane's spouse.

ABC Premiere Health Plan

MEMBER	**POLICY NUMBER**
JANE B.	WHITE HS 123456 7890

GROUP
STATE
TYPE EFFEC 01012005
EMPLOYEE-ONLY
SEND ALL BILLS TO:
ABC Premiere Health Plan
1500 Primrose Path
Flowerville, XX 12345

a. No, the card states "Employee-Only"

b. Yes, the policy number includes "S"

c. Yes, the group is "State"

d. Cannot be determined

344. From the figure, determine which entity that has purchased the insurance policy.

a. 1234567890
b. STATE
c. ABC Premiere Health Plan
d. Jane B. White

345. Bob Smith was admitted to Mercy Hospital on June 21. The physical was completed on June 23. According to CMS Conditions of Participation, which statement applies to this situation?

a. The record is not in compliance as the physical exam must be completed within 24 hours of admission.
b. The record is not in compliance as the physical exam must be completed within 48 hours of admission.
c. The record is in compliance as the physical exam must be completed within 48 hours.
d. The record is in compliance as the physical exam was completed within 72 hours of admission.

346. A clinical documentation improvement (CDI) program facilitates accurate coding and helps coders avoid:

a. NCCI edits
b. Upcoding
c. Coding without a completed face sheet
d. Assumption coding

347. Which of the following is a governmental designation by the state that is necessary for the facility to offer services?

a. Survey
b. Licensure
c. Certification
d. Accreditation

348. Reviewing claims to ensure appropriate coding for deserved payments is one method of:

a. Achieving legitimate optimization
b. Improving documentation
c. Ensuring compliance
d. Using data monitors

349. Which of the following is an example of internal medical identity theft?

a. Sue in her role as a patient registration clerk uses a patient's insurance information to see a specialist for cosmetic surgery.

b. Joe uses a patient's information obtained through hacking the healthcare facility system.

c. Joan, an ICU nurse accesses the record of the patient she is currently treating.

d. Bob introduces a virus into the facility's health information system.

350. It is the year 201X. The federal government is determined to lower the overall payments to physicians. To incur the least administrative work, which of the following elements of the physician payment system would the government reduce?

a. Conversion factor

b. RVU

c. GPCI

d. Weighted discount

351. A Joint Commission accredited organization must review their formulary annually to ensure a medication's continued:

a. Safety and dose

b. Efficiency and efficacy

c. Efficacy and safety

d. Dose and efficiency

352. Part of the coding supervisor's responsibility is to review accounts that have not been final billed due to errors. One of the accounts on the list is a same-day procedure. Upon review, the coding supervisor notices that the charge code on the bill was hard-coded. The ambulatory procedure coder added the same CPT code to the abstract. How should this error be corrected?

a. Delete the code from the CDM because it should not be there.

b. Refer the case to the chargemaster coordinator.

c. Force a final bill on the accounts since the duplication will not affect the UB-04.

d. Remove the code from the abstract and counsel the coder regarding CDM hard codes in this service.

353. In performing an internal audit for coding compliance, which of the following would be suitable case selections for auditing?

a. Infrequent diagnosis and procedure codes

b. Medical and surgical MS-DRGs by low dollar and low volume

c. Medical and surgical MS-DRGs by high dollar and high volume

d. Low-volume admission diagnoses

354. In the HHPPS system, which home healthcare services are consolidated into a single payment to home health agencies?

a. Home health aide visits, routine and nonroutine medical supplies, durable medical equipment

b. Routine and nonroutine medical supplies, durable medical equipment, medical social services

c. Nursing and therapy services, routine and nonroutine medical supplies, home health aide visits

d. Nursing and therapy services, durable medical equipment, medical social services

355. The coder assigned separate codes for individual tests when a combination code exists. This is an example of which of the following?

a. Upcoding

b. Complex coding

c. Query

d. Unbundling

356. Community Hospital implemented a clinical document improvement (CDI) program six months ago. The goal of the program was to improve clinical documentation to support quality of care, data quality, and HIM coding accuracy. Which of the following would be best to ensure that everyone understands the importance of this program?

a. Request that the CEO write a memorandum to all hospital staff

b. Give the chairperson of the CDI committee authority to fire employees who do not improve their clinical documentation

c. Include ancillary clinical staff and medical staff in the process

d. Request a letter of support from the Joint Commission

357. City Hospital's revenue cycle management (RCM) team has established the following benchmarks: (1) The value of discharged not final billed cases should not exceed two days of average daily revenue, and (2) AR days are not to exceed 60 days. The net average daily revenue is $1,000,000. What do the following data indicate about how City Hospital is meeting its benchmarks?

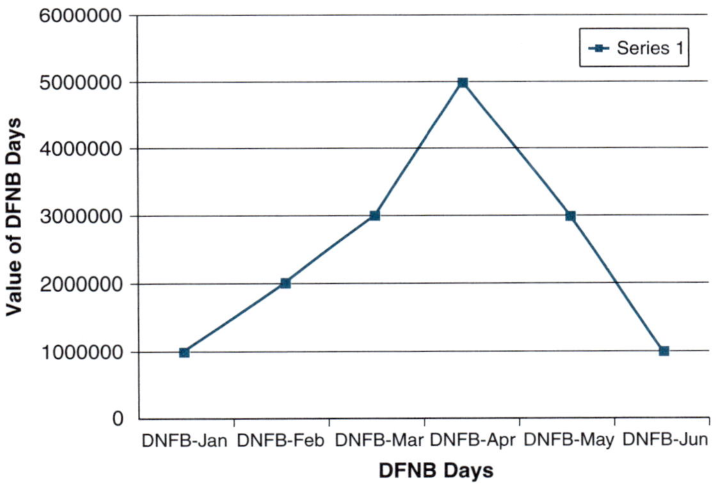

a. DNFB cases met the benchmark 100 percent of the time.

b. DNFB cases met the benchmark 75 percent of the time.

c. DNFB cases met the benchmark 50 percent of the time.

d. DNFB cases met the benchmark 25 percent of the time.

358. The accounts receivable collection cycle involves the time from:

a. Discharge to receipt of the money

b. Admission to billing the account

c. Admission to deposit in the bank

d. Billing of the account to deposit in the bank

359. In a typical acute-care setting, aging of accounts reports are monitored in which revenue cycle area?

a. Preclaims submission

b. Claims processing

c. Accounts receivable

d. Claims reconciliation or collections

360. The lead coder in the HIM department is an acknowledged coding expert and is the go-to person in the healthcare entity for coding guidance. As the HIM director you learn that she is not following proper coding guidelines and her coding practices are not compliant. As the HIM director, the best steps to take would be which of the following?

a. Report to the coder to the OIG and terminate the coder

b. Notify the compliance officer and suspend the employee

c. Review the coding errors and counsel the employee

d. Ignore the coding errors

361. To meet the definition of an inpatient rehabilitation facility (IRF), facilities must have an inpatient population with at least a specified percentage of patients with certain conditions. Which of the following conditions is counted in the definition?

a. Brain injury

b. Chronic myelogenous leukemia

c. Acute myocardial infarction

d. Cancer

362. Medicaid coverage is not identical in New Jersey, California, and Idaho. Which of the following reasons is correct?

a. Federal funds allocated to each state are based on the size of the state.

b. The program must cover infants born to Medicaid-eligible pregnant women.

c. States that offer an SCHIP program do not have a Medicaid program.

d. Medicaid allows states to maintain a unique program adapted to state residents' needs and average incomes.

363. The process in which a healthcare entity addresses the provider documentation issues of legibility, completeness, clarity, consistency, and precision is called:

a. Query process

b. Release of information process

c. Coding process

d. Case-finding process

364. What is it called when accrediting bodies such as the Joint Commission or American Osteopathic Association can survey facilities for compliance with the Medicare Conditions of Participation for hospitals instead of the government?

a. Deemed status

b. Judicial decision

c. Subpoena

d. Credentialing

365. Which of the following items are packaged under the Medicare hospital outpatient prospective payment system (OPPS)?

a. Recovery room and medical visits

b. Medical visits and supplies (other than pass-through)

c. Anesthesia and ambulance services

d. Supplies (other than pass-through) and recovery room

366. In terms of grouping and reimbursement, how are the MS-LTC-DRGs and acute-care MS-DRGs similar?

a. Relative weights

b. Based on principal diagnosis

c. Categorization of low-volume groups into quintiles

d. Classification of short-stay outliers

367. Which of the following elements is found in a charge description master?

a. ICD-10-CM code

b. Procedure or service charge

c. Patient disposition

d. Procedural service date

368. Which of the following is used to reconcile accounts in the patient accounting department?

a. Explanation of benefits

b. Medicare code editor

c. Preauthorization form

d. Fee schedule

369. Anywhere Hospital is implementing a new clinical documentation improvement (CDI) program. As part of the program, the clinical staff is educated on the components and procedures of the program. Which of the following would ***not*** be true about the CDI program?

a. The need for postdischarge queries will be eliminated.

b. Physicians will be consulted about nonspecific documentation while patients are still in-house.

c. Effective communication between clinical staff and CDI specialist is vital.

d. CDI reviewers will be on the inpatient units to review clinical documentation concurrently.

370. In a typical acute-care setting, the explanation of benefits, Medicare summary notice, and remittance advice documents (provided by the payer) are monitored in which revenue cycle area?

a. Preclaims submission

b. Claims processing

c. Accounts receivable

d. Claims reconciliation and collections

371. Which Joint Commission survey methodology involves an evaluation that follows the hospital experiences of current patients?

a. Priority focus review
b. Periodic performance review
c. Tracer methodology
d. Performance improvement

372. The health record review process and what other aspect allow for the highest level of quality in clinical documentation?

a. Training on the revenue cycle
b. Medical necessity
c. Training on basics of coding
d. Physician queries

373. The purpose of this program is to reduce improper Medicare payments and prevent future improper payments made on claims of healthcare services:

a. Medicare provider analysis and review
b. Recovery audit contractors
c. Medicare Conditions of Participation
d. Health Insurance Portability and Accountability Act

374. The following are the most common reasons for claim denials ***except***:

a. Billing noncovered services
b. Lack of medical necessity
c. Beneficiary not covered
d. Coverage not in effect for date of service

375. Charges for items that must be reported separately but are used together, such as interventional radiology imaging and injection procedures are called:

a. Insurance code mappings
b. Charge codes
c. Exploding charges
d. Revenue Codes

376. Which of the following is a characteristic of an organized medical staff as recognized by the Joint Commission?

a. Peer review activities are optional unless requested by a physician.
b. Fully licensed physicians are permitted by law to provide patient care services.
c. Delineation of clinical privileges is not necessary.
d. The medical staff is not subject to medical staff bylaws or rules, regulations, and policies, and is subject to their professional code of ethics.

377. A quality data review that is based on specific problems after an initial baseline review that has been completed in a hospital is called a(n):

a. Focused inpatient review
b. Compliance initiative
c. Internal audit
d. Concurrent review

378. With what agency may patients file a complaint if they suspect medical identity theft violations?

a. Internal Revenue Service
b. Office of Civil Rights
c. Centers for Medicare and Medicaid Services
d. Federal Trade Commission

379. A health record technician is preparing a bill for a patient who has two different third-party payers. Verification of the payers has been performed. Before either of the payers can be billed, the health record technician has to:

a. Contact the attending physician
b. Contact the patient
c. Determine which policy is primary and which is secondary
d. Determine who is the primary policy holder

380. Which of the following can be a tool for recovery audit contractors' (RAC) preparation because they outline the hospital's Medicare payment patterns compared to other hospitals in the state?

a. PEPPER
b. HITECH
c. HIPAA
d. MEDPAR

381. In the APC system, a high-cost outlier payment is paid when which of the following occurs?

a. The cost of the service is greater than the APC payment by a fixed ratio and exceeds the APC payment plus a threshold amount.
b. The LOS is greater than expected.
c. The charges for the services provided are greater than the expected payment.
d. The total cost of all the services is greater than the sum of APC payments by a fixed ratio and exceeds the sum of APC payments plus a threshold amount.

382. An internal coding audit at Community Hospital shows that the cause of improper coding is lack of proper physician documentation to support reimbursement at the appropriate level. Coders have found that coding issues result because physician documentation needs clarification. The HIM department staff has met periodically with each clinical specialty to improve communication and provide targeted education, but documentation problems still persist. Which of the following actions would be the most reliable and consistent method to improve communication and documentation?

a. Revise medical staff bylaws to include documentation requirements.
b. Suspend medical staff privileges after a specified number of documentation problems have occurred.
c. Implement a standardized physician query form so that coders can request clarification from physicians about documentation issues.
d. Allow coders to make clinical judgments in the absence of physician documentation.

383. The facility's Medicare case-mix index has dropped, although other statistical measures appear constant. The CFO suspects coding errors. What type of coding quality review should be performed?

a. Random audit

b. Focused audit

c. Compliance audit

d. External audit

384. During a recent coding audit, the coding manager identified the following error made by a coder. The coder assigned the following codes for a female patient who was admitted for stress incontinence and a urethral suspension without mesh was performed:

N39.3 Stress incontinence (female) (male)
0TUD0JZ Urethral suspension

What error was made by the coder?

N23	Unspecified renal colic
N39.3	Stress incontinence (female) (male)
R32	Unspecified urinary incontinence

Section	Body System	Root Operation	Body Part	Approach	Device	Qualifier
Medical and Surgical	Urinary System	Reposition	Urethra	Open	No Device	No Qualifier
0	T	S	D	0	Z	Z

Section	Body System	Root Operation	Body Part	Approach	Device	Qualifier
Medical and Surgical	Urinary System	Supplement	Urethra	Open	Synthetic Substitute	No Qualifier
0	T	U	D	0	J	Z

a. The coder assigned the correct diagnosis and procedure codes.

b. The coder assigned the correct diagnosis code but assigned the incorrect root operation for the procedure.

c. The coder assigned the correct procedure code but the incorrect diagnosis code.

d. The coder assigned the correct diagnosis code but selected the incorrect device character for the procedure code.

385. What is the name of the statement sent after the provider files a claim that details amounts billed by the provider, amounts approved by Medicare, amount Medicare paid, and amount the patient must pay?

a. EOB

b. MSN

c. EOMB

d. ABN

386. According to the Joint Commission, the unanticipated death of a full-term infant should be reported as a(n):

a. Sentinel event
b. Violation of clinical practice guideline
c. Unfortunate accident
d. Medical accident

387. Which of the following is the principal goal of internal auditing programs for billing and coding?

a. Increase revenues
b. Protect providers from sanctions or fines
c. Improve patient care
d. Limit unnecessary changes to the chargemaster

388. You are the coding manager and are completing a review of a new coder's work. The case facts are that the patient was treated in the emergency department for two forearm lacerations that were both repaired with simple closure. The new coder assigned one CPT code for the largest laceration. Which of the following would be the correct CPT code assignment for this case?

a. One CPT code for the largest laceration
b. Two CPT codes, one for each laceration
c. One CPT code adding the lengths of the lacerations together
d. One CPT code for the most complex closure

389. Which of the following requires financial institutions to develop written medical identity theft programs?

a. HIPAA Security Rule
b. HITECH Act
c. Fair and Accurate Credit Transactions Act
d. HIPAA Privacy and Security Rule

390. A patient is admitted to the hospital with shortness of breath and congestive heart failure. The patient undergoes intubation with mechanical ventilation. The final diagnoses documented by the attending physician are: Congestive heart failure, mechanical ventilation, and intubation. Which of the following actions should the coder take in this case?

a. Code congestive heart failure, respiratory failure, mechanical ventilation, and intubation
b. Query the attending physician as to the reason for the intubation and mechanical ventilation to add as a secondary diagnosis
c. Query the attending physician about the adding the symptom of shortness of breath as a secondary diagnosis
d. Code shortness of breath, congestive heart failure, mechanical ventilation, and intubation

391. Data-mining efforts of recovery audit contractors (RAC) allow them to deny payments without ever reviewing a health record based on the information they gather without having access to the record. Which of the following would be an example of a potential denial based on information the RAC contractor would have without the health record?

a. A coder assigning the wrong DRG for a patient
b. Billing for two colonoscopies on the same day for the same Medicare beneficiary
c. An inaccurate principal diagnosis
d. A principal procedure code

392. You are the coding manager and are completing a review of a new coder's work. The case facts are that the patient was admitted for the treatment of dehydration secondary to chemotherapy for primary liver cancer. The new coder sequenced the principal diagnosis as liver carcinoma. Which of the following would be the correct principal diagnosis?

a. Liver carcinoma
b. Admission for chemotherapy
c. Dehydration
d. Complication of chemotherapy

393. The Medicare programs that encourage patients to review provider bills carefully and to report any discrepancies to the Secretary of HHS are called:

a. Beneficiary incentive programs
b. OIG work plans
c. Compliance initiatives
d. Operation Restore Trust programs

394. The most recent coding audit has revealed a tendency to miss secondary diagnoses that would have increased the reimbursement for the case. Which of the following strategies would be most likely to correct this problem in the long term?

a. Focused reviews on changes in MS-DRGs
b. Facility top 10 to 15 DRGs by volume and charges
c. Contracting with a larger consulting firm to do audits and education
d. Development and implementation of a CDI program

Domain 5 *Leadership*

395. Which of the following are alternate work scheduling techniques?

a. Compressed workweek, open systems, and job sharing
b. Flextime, telecommuting, and compressed workweek
c. Telecommuting, open systems, and flextime
d. Flextime, outsourcing, compressed workweek

396. The time required to recoup the cost of an investment is called the:

a. Accounting rate of return
b. Budget cycle
c. Payback period
d. Depreciation

397. Violation of the AHIMA Code of Ethics triggers:

a. Automatic loss of AHIMA credentials
b. Disciplinary actions and a fine
c. A review by peers with potential disciplinary actions
d. Nothing because a violation of ethics is not a big deal

398. Change management includes:

a. Identifying problems
b. Being available to listen to staff
c. Redesigning processes
d. Educating staff on new processes

399. One of the most common issues that healthcare organizations fail to do well in the strategic process is:

a. Develop a vision
b. Develop strategies
c. Execute the implementation plan
d. Communicate the plan

400. The percent of antibiotics administered immediately prior to open reduction and internal fixation (ORIF) surgeries or the percent of deliveries accomplished by cesarean section are examples of what type of performance measure?

a. Outcome measure
b. Data measure
c. Process measure
d. System measure

Use the following information for questions 401 and 402:

> At the end of March, the HIM department has a YTD payroll budget of $100,000. The actual YTD amount paid is $95,000 because a coder resigned in February. For the past two months, the position has been filled through outsourcing. Therefore, the actual YTD amount for consulting services is $5,000, although no money was budgeted for consulting services. The reporting threshold for variances is 4 percent. The fiscal year-end is December.

401. What is the best description of the consulting services variance?

a. Favorable, permanent
b. Unfavorable, permanent
c. Favorable, temporary
d. Unfavorable, temporary

402. Which one of the variances will the HIM director be required to explain?

a. Only the consulting services variance
b. Only the payroll variance
c. Both the payroll and consulting services variances
d. Neither because the two variances cancel each other out

403. The performance standard "File 50 to 60 records per hour" is an example of a:

a. Quality standard
b. Quantity standard
c. Joint Commission standard
d. Compliance standard

404. What could an analysis of a flowchart identify?

a. Productivity levels
b. Customer needs
c. Key performance measures
d. Redundancies in a process

405. When implementing health information management training, determining who needs to be trained, who should do the training, how much training is required, and how the training will be accomplished is the responsibility of:

a. The vendor
b. Information systems
c. Health information management
d. The implementation team

406. Sandy is coder but would like to be a privacy officer one day. Joan, the privacy officer at her hospital, has agreed to help Sandy on her career path. Joan has suggested that Sandy begin to look at master's degree programs and has taken her to a local association meeting where she can begin to network with other privacy officers. This is an example of:

a. Continuing education
b. Job rotation
c. Mentoring
d. Succession planning

407. Systems thinking focuses on an understanding of which of the following?

a. The relationships among parts and processes of the healthcare entity and how they work together
b. The operational level of strategy
c. How successful leader traits develop and may be overused
d. The formulation of envisioning used by the leader to develop esprit

408. The focus of conflict management is:

a. Getting personal counseling for the parties involved
b. Separating the parties involved so that they do not have to work together
c. Working with the parties involved to find a mutually acceptable solution
d. Bringing disciplinary action against one party or the other

409. A coding service had 400 discharged records to code in March. The service coded 200 within 3 days, 100 within 5 days, 50 within 8 days, and 50 within 10 days. The average turnaround time (TAT) for coding in March was:

a. 3 days
b. 5 days
c. 6.5 days
d. 9 days

410. Coders at Medical Center Hospital are expected to do a high volume of coding. Their department also includes a clerical support person who handles phone calls, pulls and files records to be coded, and maintains productivity logs. An abstract clerk enters coded data into the health information system. This is an example of ________ work division.

a. Parallel
b. Unit
c. Serial
d. Serial unit

411. The leader of the coding performance improvement team wants all team members to clearly understand the coding process. What tool could help accomplish this objective?

a. Flowchart
b. Force-field analysis
c. Pareto chart
d. Scatter diagram

412. What kind of planning addresses long-term needs and sets comprehensive plans of action?

a. Tactical
b. Operational
c. Strategic
d. Administrative

413. All variances (as related to accounting) should be labeled as either:

a. Good or bad
b. Favorable or unfavorable
c. Positive or negative
d. Over budget or under budget

414. This type of performance measure indicates the result of the performance or nonperformance of a function or process.

a. Outcome measure
b. Data measure
c. Process measure
d. System measure

415. Employees, physicians, and other stakeholders are invited to town hall meetings, receive newsletters and e-mail, and can check social media for the status of the EHR implementation project. This is an example of good:

a. Management
b. Project planning
c. Communication
d. Marketing

416. Capital budgeting differs from operational budgeting in what manner?

a. It is generally limited to one fiscal year.
b. It involves high-dollar purchases and multiple-year projects.
c. It is usually started after completing the operating budget.
d. It is for purchases other than equipment.

417. The statement "Coding of inpatient records must be completed at a 98 percent accuracy rate" is an example of a:

a. Goal
b. Vision statement
c. Qualitative standard
d. Quantitative standard

418. The performance standard "Complete five birth certificates per hour" is an example of a:

a. Quality standard
b. Quantity standard
c. Joint Commission standard
d. Compliance standard

419. How are employee performance standards used?

a. To communicate performance expectations

b. To assign daily work

c. To describe the elements of a job

d. To prepare a job advertisement

420. The predefined process icon 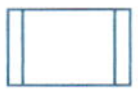 is used in flowcharting to indicate:

a. A process in which actions are being performed by humans

b. A point in the process at which participants must evaluate the status of the process

c. Formal procedures that participants are expected to carry out the same way every time

d. A point in the process at which the participants must record data in paper-based or computer-based formats

421. An analysis of a company's liquidity attempts to measure the company's ability to:

a. Meet long-term debt payments

b. Pay dividends each year

c. Meet current debt payments

d. Make a profit

422. When an effective leader provides employees with information, responsibility, authority, and trust, this is called:

a. Empowerment

b. Promotion

c. Vision

d. Delegation

423. Generally, substantial performance by one party to a contract will obligate the other party:

a. To perform their contractual obligations

b. Not to perform their contractual obligations

c. To void the contract

d. To invalidate the contract

424. Annual renewal of fire safety and disaster preparedness are topics that may be addressed best through training known as:

a. Job rotation

b. Customer service

c. In-service education

d. Pay for performance

425. Which of the following would be considered a discriminatory practice in the employment setting?

a. Denial of employment based on criminal record.

b. Screening out an applicant who does not meet the minimum qualifications for the position.

c. Denial of employment based on religion.

d. Hiring a person based on vision of the healthcare entity.

426. What actions might be taken to reduce the risks of groupthink?

a. High cohesion without interaction with outside groups
b. Monitoring the degree of consensus and disagreement
c. The leader states his or her opinion early to influence the rest of the group
d. Limit organizational controls

427. Which of the following is considered a viable solution to a staff recruitment problem for coding and transcription shortages?

a. Delegation
b. Job distribution
c. Overtime
d. Telecommuting

428. Under the Americans with Disabilities Act, employees receive protection with respect to their job duties if they are able to perform the necessary functions of a job:

a. As the job exists
b. With reasonable accommodations
c. With changes to the work arrangements
d. While sharing the job with another employee

429. Which of the following are attributes of both projects and daily operations?

a. Defined start dates
b. Roles and responsibilities
c. Set budgets or costs
d. Defined finish dates

430. At Community Health Services, each budget cycle provides the opportunity to continue or discontinue services based on available resources so that every department or activity must be justified and prioritized annually in order to effectively allocate resources. Community Health uses what type of operational budget?

a. Activity-based
b. Fixed
c. Flexible
d. Zero-based

431. In project management, what is a work breakdown structure?

a. Manages the risks of the project
b. Hierarchical list of the project tasks
c. Document that defines team roles and responsibilities
d. List of project scope changes

432. Work products that must be produced as a result of a project are referred to as:

a. Materials
b. Resources
c. Sponsors
d. Deliverables

433. Ethical obligation to the ________ include advocating change when patterns or system problems are not in the best interest of the patients, reporting violation of practice standards to the proper authorities.

a. Employer

b. Self, peers, and professional associations

c. AHIMA organization

d. Public

434. Net income is defined as the:

a. Difference between revenue and expenses

b. Difference between total assets and total liabilities

c. Difference between revenue and total liabilities

d. Difference between net assets and expenses

435. The manual input icon 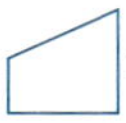 is used in flowcharting to indicate:

a. A process when in which are being performed by a computer

b. A point in the process at which participants must evaluate the status of the process

c. Formal procedures that participants are expected to carry out the same way every time

d. A point in the process at which the participants must record data in paper-based or computer-based formats

436. Which of the following is a characteristic of strategic management?

a. Shifting the balance of power to the employees

b. Creating a plan to avoid change within the healthcare entity

c. A description of specific implementation plans

d. A plan to improve the healthcare entity's fit with the external world

437. A physician who provides care in a healthcare facility, is not employed by the healthcare entity and therefore not under the direct control or supervision of another, and is personally responsible for his or her negligent acts and carries his or her own professional liability insurance is considered a(n) ________ to the healthcare entity.

a. Agent

b. Independent contractor

c. Supervisor

d. Vendor

438. Which financial statement reflects the extent to which a healthcare entity's revenues exceed its expenses?

a. Balance sheet

b. Statement of cash flows

c. Statement of retained earnings

d. Income statement

439. The financial statement that communicates the financial position of an organization at a certain point in time is called the:

a. Income statement

b. Balance sheet

c. Statement of cash flows

d. Statement of retained earnings

440. What is the process of finding, soliciting, and attracting new employees called?

a. Recruitment

b. Retention

c. Orientation

d. Hiring

441. Which of the following statements describes a critical skill for a strategic manager?

a. Ability to change direction quickly

b. Ability to deliver results on budget

c. Ability to envision relationships between trends and opportunities

d. Ability to design jobs and match peoples' skills to them

442. Which of the following best categorizes the group of adopters who comprise the backbone of the organization, are conventional and deliberate in their decisions, and form a bridge with other adopter categories?

a. Innovators

b. Early adopters

c. Early majority

d. Late majority

443. When a computer-assisted coding product was installed at Community Memorial Hospital, coders initially found the new system overwhelming and were frustrated because their productivity decreased significantly. This experience represents the first stages of a(n):

a. Incentive system

b. Flex system

c. In-service program

d. Learning curve

444. Which tool is used to determine the most critical areas for training and education for a group of employees?

a. Performance evaluation

b. Needs analysis

c. Orientation assessment

d. Job specification

445. Which of the following is a statement made by one party to induce another party to enter into a contract?

a. *Ultra vires*

b. Warranty

c. Agreement

d. Indemnification

446. Use of a variety of content delivery methods to accommodate different types of learners is called:

a. Blended learning

b. Programmed learning

c. Classroom learning

d. Online learning

447. The correct sequence of steps when evaluating an ethical problem is:

a. Who are the stakeholders, what are the options, what is the decision, what justifies the choice,, determine the facts, and identify prevention options

b. What are the options, what is the decision, who are the stakeholders, what justifies the choice, identify prevention options, and determine the facts

c. Determine the facts, what are the options, what is the decision, what justifies the choice, who are the stakeholders, and identify prevention options

d. Determine the facts, who are the stakeholders, what are the options, what is the decision, what justifies the choice, and identify prevention options

448. A strategy map can be a useful tool because it:

a. Provides a record of progress toward goals

b. Provides a visual framework for integrating strategies

c. Enables others to better understand the vision underlying change

d. Enables assignment of essential resources to executing the plan

449. Determining costs associated with EHR hardware and software acquisition, implementation, and ongoing maintenance represents which type of analysis?

a. Benefits realization study

b. Goal-setting exercise

c. Cost–benefit feasibility study

d. Productivity improvement study

450. In the following figure, identify the component of the project plan labeled as D.

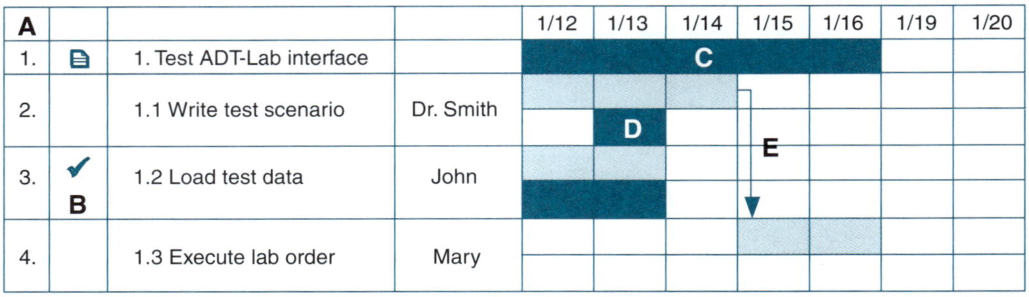

a. Row numbers

b. Task completed

c. Task progress

d. Dependency

451. The three levels of communication important to successful EHR implementation among internal stakeholders include all of the following ***except***:

a. Between executive leadership, stakeholders, and vendors

b. Between stakeholders and standard-setting organizations

c. From stakeholder to stakeholder

d. Between executive leadership and internal stakeholders

452. The performance standard "Transcribe 1,500 lines per day" is an example of a:

a. Quality standard

b. Quantity standard

c. Joint Commission standard

d. Compliance standard

453. Joe is hired as a floater in a health information department to fill in wherever help is needed. He learns the jobs of several employees. This is an example of:

a. Outsourcing

b. Physical training

c. Cross-training

d. Performance evaluation

454. Heather and Jim are both coders at Medical Center Hospital. The hospital allows them to set their own hours as long as one of them is in the office between 9:00 a.m. and 3:00 p.m. so they are accessible to physicians. This kind of work arrangement is called:

a. Telecommuting

b. Compressed workweek

c. Outsourcing

d. Flextime

455. Which of the following would ***not*** be included in a healthcare entity's strategic profile?

a. Nature of its threats and opportunities

b. Nature of its customers or users

c. Nature of its market segments

d. Nature of its geographic markets

456. If parties to a contract agree to hold each other harmless for each other's actions or inactions, this is referred to as a(n):

a. Indemnification

b. Liability

c. Offer

d. Warranty

457. What is the first step in a successful departmental training and development plan?

a. Designing the curriculum

b. Selecting the delivery methods

c. Determining the latest hot topic

d. Performing a needs analysis

458. The leaders of a healthcare entity are expected to select an entity-wide performance improvement approach and to clearly define how all levels of the entity will monitor and address improvement issues. The Joint Commission requires ongoing data collection that might require possible improvement for which of the following areas?

a. Operative and other invasive procedures, medication management, and blood and blood product use

b. Blood and blood product use, medication management, and appointment to the board of directors

c. Medication management, marketing strategy, and blood use

d. Operative and other invasive procedures, appointments to the board of directors, and restraint and seclusion use

459. Which of the following is a common outcome of conflict in the workplace?

a. Increased morale

b. Increased retention

c. Feeling of safety

d. Decreased productivity

460. Which work measurement tool uses random sample observations to obtain information about the performance of an entire department?

a. Performance measurement

b. Work distribution

c. Work sampling

d. Performance controls

Answer Key

Exam 1 Answers

Domain 1

1. **d** Transfer records are created whenever a patient is transferred from one facility to another. The transfer record contains a summary of the care provided in the facility from which the patient is being transferred as well as the reason for transfer. Transfer records are important to the continuum of care because they document communication between caregivers in multiple settings (Russo 2013a, 225).

2. **a** The chief complaint or reason for the visit is the nature and duration of the symptoms that caused the patient's illness and caused the patient to seek medical attention as stated in the patient's own words. In this scenario the patient came in complaining of abdominal pain, so this is the chief complaint (Rossiter 2013, 502).

3. **b** Data quality needs to be consistent. A difference in the birth dates provides a good example of how the lack of consistency can lead to problems (Sharp and Madlock-Brown 2016, 197).

4. **c** Coded data is data that is translated into standard nomenclature of classification so that it may be aggregated, analyzed, and compared (AHIMA 2014, 29).

5. **d** Authentication means to prove authorship and can be done in several ways. Methods of electronically signing documentation include a digital signature (a digitized image of a signature), a biometric identifier such as fingerprint or retinal scan, or a code or password. In today's health record, electronic signatures are used more frequently as more documents in the record are produced by, and remain in, the electronic health record system rather than becoming part of the paper record. The physician assistant and charge nurse cannot authenticate the physician's entry in lieu of the physician as it is the physician's documentation. Likewise, having the HIM clerk use a physician's signature stamp is not an accepted method of authentication (Reynolds and Sharp 2016, 124).

6. **a** Basic clinical data, such as the type of surgery or reason for the visit, is collected and recorded during the intake process. From this, the treating or admitting physician can provide the patient's preliminary diagnosis and the reason the patient is seeking treatment. Accurate clinical data collection is important because it becomes the basis of care plans and helps determine medical necessity (Fahrenholz 2013b, 77).

7. **a** Resident assessment protocols (RAPs) form a critical link to decisions about care planning and provide guidance on how to synthesize assessment information within a comprehensive assessment. The triggers target conditions for additional assessment and review, as warranted by Minimum Data Set (MDS) item responses. The RAPs guidelines help facility staff evaluate triggered conditions (CMS 2010; James 2013b, 538).

8. **d** The health information management (HIM) director is generally responsible for implementing the retention program; however, other individuals may be charged with the shared responsibility of implementing the program in some facilities. Some facilities establish a task force to oversee the record retention program, and this is sometimes chaired by the HIM professional. The steps in developing a record retention program include: conducting an inventory of the facility's records, determining the format and location of record storage, assigning each record a retention period, and destroying records that are no longer needed (Reynolds and Sharp 2016, 133–135).

9. **b** The principal function of the health record is to serve as the repository of clinical documentation relevant to the care of individual patients. The principal functions are related to specific healthcare encounters between providers and patients (Fahrenholz 2013b, 75).

10. **d** Clinical information is the basis for uniform data sets. The clinical information in the patient's record is primarily used to treat the patient. However, when clinical information from many patient records is combined, a data set can facilitate the comparison of patient information from multiple sources (Russo 2013a, 295).

11. **c** The documentation that comprises the legal health record (LHR) may physically exist in separate and multiple paper-based or electronic systems. This complicates the process of pulling the entire legal record together in response to authorized requests to produce the complete patient record. Once the LHR is defined, it is best practice to create a health record matrix that identifies and tracks the physical location of each paper document and the source of each electronic document that constitutes the LHR. In addition to defining the content of the LHR, it is best practice to establish a policy statement on the maintenance of it (Rinehart-Thompson 2016, 61).

12. **b** The content of the emergency health record should generally include the time and means of arrival, treatment rendered, and instructions at discharge. Facilities are required to do a pertinent history, including the chief complaint and onset of illness or injury but not a complete medical history of the patient (Giannangelo 2016, 116–117).

13. **d** All ICD-10-PCS codes must be seven characters, and a character cannot be left blank. If a value does not exist for a given character, the Z is used as the value (Kuehn and Jorwic 2017, 4).

14. **d** The unique identifier in the patient table is the patient number. It is unique to each patient. Patient last name, first name, and date of birth can be shared with other patients, but the identifier will not (Biedermann and Dolezel 2017, 189).

15. **b** The Minimum Data Set (MDS) is a component of the resident assessment instrument (RAI) and is used to collect information about the resident's risk factors and to plan the ongoing care and treatment of the resident in the long-term care facility (James 2013b, 536).

16. **c** Ownership of the health record is generally granted to the healthcare provider who generates the record. Since the record serves as both a medical document and as a legal document that provides proof of care, it is the business record of the healthcare provider (Fahrenholz 2013a, 26–27).

17. **b** When tasked with assessing or managing data quality, an HIM professional must first understand who the data consumers are and what their needs are. This involves making a list of all of the internal and external consumers. Assessing the needs of data consumers is challenging; a good data manager would ask the data consumer how they use the data rather than what their needs are. The data manager must take a controlled and careful approach to collecting data for consumer needs. It will be impossible for the data manager to meet all the needs of all of the data consumers (Biedermann and Dolezel 2017, 167–168).

18. **c** The Subjective, Objective, Assessment, Plan (SOAP) notes are part of the problem-oriented medical records (POMR) approach most commonly used by physicians and other healthcare professionals. SOAP notes are intended to improve the quality and continuity of client services by enhancing communication among healthcare professionals (Russo 2013b, 303–305).

19. **a** The anemia D50.0 was not specified as acute and would be sequenced first based on principal diagnosis guidelines followed by the code N93.8 for the dysfunctional uterine bleeding (Schraffenberger and Palkie 2017, 91).

20. **d** Financial data includes details about the patient's occupation, employer, and insurance coverage and is collected at the time of treatment. Healthcare providers use this data to complete claims forms that will be submitted to third-party payers (Fahrenholz 2013b, 76).

21. **a** Entity relationship modeling is a type of conceptual modeling. Conceptual models are abstract and encourage high-level problem structuring; they help establish a common ground for communication between users and developers. The entity-relationship diagram (ERD) was developed to depict relational database structures (Sharp and Madlock-Brown 2016, 183)

22. **c** The closed reduction of the fracture is coded because it is the main procedure. The laceration repair is also coded. A–59 modifier would need to be added to the laceration code to indicate a distinct procedural service for billing purposes. When more than one classification of wound repair is performed, all codes are reported with the code for the most complicated procedure listed first (Kuehn 2017, 26, 110).

23. **b** A many-to-many relationship occurs only in a data model developed at the conceptual level. In this case, the relationship between PATIENTS and CONSULTING PHYSICIANS is many-to-many. For each instance of PATIENT, there could be many instances of CONSULTING PHYSICIAN because patients can be seen by more than one consulting physician. For each instance of CONSULTING PHYSICIAN, there could be many PATIENTS because the physician sees many patients (Sayles and Trawick 2014, 56).

24. **b** The root operation performed was division—cutting into a body part without drawing fluids or gases from the body part in order to separate or transect a body part. The intent of the operation was to separate the femur, so 0Q860ZZ is the correct code. The Section is Medical and Surgical—character 0; Body System is Lower Bones—character Q; Root Operation is Division—character 8; Body Part is Upper Femur, Right—character 6; Approach is Open—character 0; No Device—character Z; and No Qualifier—character Z (Kuehn and Jorwic 2017, 21–23, 99).

25. **b** Authorship is the origin of recorded information that is attributed to a specific individual or entity. Electronic tools make it easier to copy and paste documentation from one record to another or to pull information forward from a previous visit, someone else's records, or other sources either intentionally or inadvertently. The ability to copy and paste entries leads to a record where a clinician may, upon signing the documentation, unwittingly swear to the accuracy and comprehensiveness of substantial amounts of duplicated, inapplicable, misleading, or erroneous information (Russo 2013b, 339).

26. **c** An author is a person or system who originates or creates information that becomes part of the record. Each author must be granted permission by the healthcare entity to make such entries. Not all users will be granted authorship rights into all areas of the electronic health record (EHR). The individual must have the credentials required by state and federal laws to be granted the right to document observations and facts related to the provision of healthcare services. Authentication is a process by which a user (a person or entity) who authored an EHR entry or document is seeking to validate that they are responsible for the data contained within it (Biedermann and Dolezel 2017, 442–443).

27. **b** The coding professional's first responsibility is to ensure the accuracy of coded data. To this end, AHIMA has established a code of professional ethics by which coders must abide (Hazelwood and Venable 2016, 204).

28. **b** The American Health Information Management Association (AHIMA) recommends that records be destroyed in such a way that the information cannot possibly be reconstructed. The destruction should be documented, and the documentation should include the following: date of destruction, method of destruction (shredding, burning, or other means), description of the disposed record series of numbers or items, inclusive dates covered, a statement that the records were destroyed in the normal course of business, and the signatures of the individuals supervising and witnessing the destruction. AHIMA further recommends that facilities maintain destruction certification documents permanently. Such certificates may be required as evidence that records were destroyed in the regular course of business. When facilities fail to apply destruction policies uniformly or when destruction is contrary to policy, courts may allow a jury to infer that the facility destroyed its records to hide evidence (Reynolds and Sharp 2016, 137).

29. **b** The data dictionary may also control if a mask is used and if so, what form it takes. The Social Security number of 123456789 could be entered and it appears in the system as 123-45-6789. The use of the mask tells the database what format to use to display the number (Sayles and Trawick 2014, 53–54).

30. **b** The primary key (PK) for PATIENT, PATIENT_MRN, is repeated in VISIT, as is the PK for CLINIC, CLINIC_ID. These keys are called foreign keys (FK) in the VISIT table. Foreign keys allow relationships between tables. By having the foreign keys in VISIT, the information in PATIENT and CLINIC is linked through the VISIT table (Johns 2015, 128–129).

31. **c** Data governance is an emerging practice in the healthcare industry. Decision making and authority over data-related matters is data governance. It is clear that any industry as reliant on data as healthcare needs a plan for managing this asset (Biedermann and Dolezel 2017, 163).

32. **b** Metadata are often referred to as "data about data." Metadata are structured information used to increase the effective use of data. One of the most familiar types of metadata is used to describe data in databases. Data element name, data type, and field length are examples of this kind of metadata (Johns 2016, 82–83).

33. **b** The patient was admitted for diabetic cataract. There is a causal relationship given between the diabetes and the cataract, so E11.36 would be assigned. This follows the UHDDS guidelines for principal diagnosis selection. The correct root operation is replacement because the intraocular lens was inserted at the time of the cataract extraction. Replacement is putting in or on biological or synthetic material that physically takes the place or function of all or a portion of a body part (Schraffenberger and Palkie 2017, 91, 180–181; Kuehn and Jorwic 2017, 130–131).

34. **d** Structured data commonly refer to data that are organized and easy to retrieve and to interpret by traditional databases and data models. The data elements in a patient's automated laboratory order, or result, are coded and alphanumeric. Their fields are predefined and limited. In other words, the type of data is discrete, and the format of this data is structured (Johns 2016, 83).

35. **b** The Joint Commission has established a cautious quality approach to the use of abbreviations in all its accredited organizations. To comply, every healthcare organization should strive to limit or eliminate the use of abbreviations by developing an organization-specific abbreviation list so that only those abbreviations approved by the organization are used. When more than one meaning for an approved abbreviation exists, an organization should choose only one meaning or context in which the abbreviation is to be used (Rinehart-Thompson 2017c, 186–187).

36. **a** The documentation that comprises the legal health record (LHR) may physically exist in separate and multiple paper-based or electronic systems. This complicates the process of pulling the entire legal record together in response to authorized requests to produce the complete patient record. Once the LHR is defined, it is best practice to create a health record matrix that identifies and tracks the physical location of each paper document and the source of each electronic document that constitutes the LHR. In addition to defining the content of the LHR, it is best practice to establish a policy statement on the maintenance of it (Rinehart-Thompson 2016, 60).

37. **a** For the purposes of mapping, the term coding system is used very broadly to include classification, terminology, and other data representation systems. Mapping is necessary as health information systems and their use evolves in order to link disparate systems and data sets. Any data map will include a source and a target. The source is the code or data set from which the map originates (Biedermann and Dolezel 2017, 155).

38. **c** Aggregate data are used to develop information about groups of patients (Sharp and Madlock-Brown 2016, 170).

39. **d** The clinical documentation that is entered into the patient record as text is not as easily automated due to the unstructured nature of the information. Unstructured clinical information includes notes written by physicians and other practitioners who treat the patient, dictated and transcribed reports, and legal forms such as consents and advance directives (Biedermann and Dolezel 2017, 84).

40. **c** The continued need or requirement to use paper in conjunction with an electronic health record (EHR) is known as a hybrid record. These records are the most difficult to manage because what is in paper and what is electronic may be constantly changing while the organization will have to comply with the regulations for both paper records and EHRs (Biedermann and Dolezel 2017, 264).

41. **c** Except in emergency situations, every surgical patient's chart must include a report of a complete history and physical conducted no more than seven days before the surgery is to be performed (Russo 2013a, 238).

Domain 2

42. **c** The concept of legal health records was created to describe the data, documents, reports, and information that comprise the formal business record(s) of any healthcare organization that are to be utilized during legal proceedings. Understanding legal health records requires knowledge of not only what comprises business records used as legal health records, but also the processes as well as the physical and electronic systems used to manage these records (Biedermann and Dolezel 2017, 424).

43. **d** An audit trail is a chronological set of computerized records that provides evidence of a computer system utilization (log-ins and log-outs, file accesses) used to determine security violations (Sandefer 2016a, 366).

44. **d** Unless the employer has allowed for such exclusion, it is appropriate that a patient's family history of cancer be reported to the employer. In this case the patient is being treated or examined at the request of the employer so the employer is a business associate of the clinic (Rinehart-Thompson 2017d, 211).

45. **a** This situation must be corrected. The privacy officer should complete a process flow and identify the areas where a breakdown in the process is resulting in a complaint of mailing the report to the wrong patient. It is important for the covered entity to take as many precautions as possible to ensure compliance by its workforce. Training is necessary in this situation to mitigate this type of error (Rinehart-Thompson 2017e, 255–256).

46. **c** Virtual private network (VPN) uses a secure tunnel through a public network, usually the Internet, to connect remote sites or users. Security procedures include firewalls, encryption, and server authentication (Amatayakul 2017, 335).

47. **d** Privileged communication is a legal concept designed to protect the confidentiality between two parties and is usually delineated by state law (Brodnik 2017a, 7).

48. **b** Role-based access control (RBAC) is a control system in which access decisions are based on the roles of individual users as part of an organization (Theodos 2017, 270).

49. **c** As important as firewalls are to the overall security of health information systems, they cannot protect a system from all types of attacks (Sandefer 2016a, 366).

50. **b** HIPAA requires the implementation of policies and procedures for the removal of hardware and electronic media that contain ePHI into and out of a facility. There are four implementation specifications within this standard: disposal, media reuse, accountability, and data backup and storage. In this case the organization did not follow policies for the removal of hardware and electronic media (Theodos 2017, 276).

51. **c** The Privacy Rule uses six years as the period for which Privacy Rule-related documents must be retained. The six-year time frame refers to the latter of the following: the date the document was created or the last effective date of the document. Such documents include policies and procedures, the notice of privacy practices (NPP), complaint dispositions, and other actions, activities, and designations that must be documented per Privacy Rule requirements (Rinehart-Thompson 2017e, 257).

52. **b** When obtaining consent for surgery, the surgeon is the healthcare provider who would discuss the consent for treatment with the patient. The basic elements of an informed surgical consent should include the purpose of the proposed procedure, any risks associated with the procedure, and if noninvasive treatment alternatives might be considered (Theodos 2017, 141).

53. **d** Corporate negligence is a legal doctrine that was established by a judicial decision handed down in the 1965 court case *Darling v. Charleston Community Hospital*. The court in this case ruled specifically that hospital governing boards have a duty to institute a means to evaluate and council medical staff who personally perform services on a patient that results in harm due to unreasonable risk. Hospitals may be held liable when a member of the medical staff fails to meet established standards of patient care (Pozgar 2012; Fahrenholz 2013b, 88–89).

54. **c** The National Practitioner Data Bank was created to collect information on the legal actions (both civil and criminal) taken against licensed healthcare providers (Shaw and Carter 2015, 346–347).

55. **c** The covered entity may require the individual to make an amendment request in writing and provide a rationale for it. Such a process must be communicated in advance to the individual through the organization's notice of privacy practices. Therefore, an individual cannot review his or her physical record without an authorized HIM staff member present to maintain the integrity of the record (Rinehart-Thompson 2017e, 245–246).

56. **c** Privacy is the quality or state of being hidden from, or undisturbed by, the observation or activities of other persons. It is also freedom from unauthorized intrusion. In healthcare-related contexts, privacy is the right of a patient to control disclosure of personal information (Brodnik 2017a, 6–7).

57. **c** Competent adults have a general right to consent to or refuse medical treatment. If an adult has a sound mind or did when he or she created a living will, this patient has the right to refuse treatment (Klaver 2017c, 154–155).

58. **c** Treatment, payment, and healthcare operations (45 CFR 164.501)—collectively referred to as TPO—are functions of a covered entity (CE) that are necessary for the CE to successfully conduct business. It is not the intent of the Privacy Rule to impose onerous rules that hinder a CE's functions. Therefore, many of the Privacy Rule's requirements are relaxed or removed where PHI is needed for purposes of TPO (Rinehart-Thompson 2017d, 216).

59. **d** Implied consent refers to consent for medical treatment that is communicated through a person's conduct or some other means besides words. Implied consent includes emergency situations where an individual may be unconscious or otherwise lacks capacity to communicate consent. In these cases, consent is implied by the law rather than the patient's words or conduct (Klaver 2017c, 140).

60. **c** A facility may maintain a facility directory of patients being treated. HIPAA's Privacy Rule permits the facility to maintain in its directory the following information about an individual if the individual has not objected: name, location in the facility, and condition described in general terms. This information may be disclosed to persons who ask for the individual by name (Rinehart-Thompson 2017d, 227).

61. **b** Administrative safeguards are people-focused and include requirements such as training and assignment of an individual responsible for security (Sayles and Trawick 2014, 208).

62. **c** The federal government act that developed healthcare standards governing electronic data interchange and data security is the Health Insurance Portability and Accountability Act of 1996 (Brinda and Watters 2016, 307).

63. **b** Deidentified information is information from which personal characteristics have been removed and that, as a result, neither identifies nor provides a reasonable basis to believe it could identify an individual (Rinehart-Thompson 2017d, 214).

64. **d** The Workforce Security Standard requires the organization to ensure that those with a legitimate need to access information are able to do so while at the same time ensuring that those workforce members who do not have a legitimate need to that information are prevented from gaining access. The three specifications include: authorization and supervision, workforce clearance procedures, and termination procedures. Concept supervision is not one of the three specifications (Biedermann and Dolezel 2017, 384–385).

65. **c** Generally, if the patient is a minor at the time of treatment or hospitalization but has reached the age of majority at the time the authorization for access or disclosure of information is signed, the patient's authorization is legally required (Brodnik 2017b, 343–344).

66. **c** The HIPAA Privacy Rule provides patients with significant rights that allow them to have some measure of control over their health information. As long as state laws or regulations or the physician does not state otherwise, competent adult patients have the right to access their health record (Rinehart-Thompson 2017d, 224–225).

67. **c** The signature of the attending physician, next of kin, and insurance are not necessary on a HIPAA Complaint Authorization form. The notice of privacy practices informs a patient how and when PHI can be released. If a particular use of information is not covered in the notice of privacy practices, the patient must sign an authorization form specific to the additional disclosure before his or her information can be released (Brinda and Watters 2016, 313–314).

68. **b** One of the most fundamental terms in the Privacy Rule is protected health information (PHI), defined as "individually identifiable health information that is transmitted by electronic media, maintained in electronic media, or transmitted or maintained in any other form or medium" (45 CFR 160.103). To meet the individually identifiable element of PHI, information must meet all three portions of a three-part test. (1) It must either identify the person or provide a reasonable basis to believe the person could be identified from the information given. (2) It must relate to one's past, present, or future physical or mental health condition; the provision of healthcare; or payment for the provision of healthcare. (3) It must be held or transmitted by a covered entity or its business associate. An individual's license plate is an identifier (Rinehart-Thompson 2017d, 213).

69. **b** Those who choose to destroy the original health record may do so within weeks, months, or years of scanning. If the record was destroyed according to guidelines for destruction and no scanned record exists, the certificate of destruction should be presented in lieu of the record (Reynolds and Sharp 2016, 137).

70. **a** The Privacy Rule provides patients an opportunity to agree or object to specific types of disclosure. These do not require a written authorization; verbal authorization is acceptable. However, communication with the patient regarding these types of disclosures and the patient's decision should be documented in the health record or other appropriate manner of documentation (Brinda and Watters 2016, 317).

71. **c** Hospitals strive to keep incident reports confidential, and in some states, incident reports are protected under statutes protecting quality improvement studies and activities. Incident reports themselves should not be considered a part of the health record. Because the staff member mentioned in the record that an incident report was completed, it will likely be discoverable as the health record is already a discoverable document (Rinehart-Thompson 2016, 72).

72. **c** The Office of Civil Rights of the Department of Health and Human Services has been given responsibility for the oversight and enforcement of the HIPAA regulations (Biedermann and Dolezel 2017, 352).

73. **b** For fundraising activities that benefit the covered entity (CE) 45 CFR 164.514 [f] permits the covered entity (CE) to use or disclose to a business associate or an institutionally related foundation, without authorization, demographic information and dates of healthcare provided to an individual. The CE must inform individuals on its notice of privacy practices (NPP) that PHI may be used for this purpose. If a fundraising activity targets individuals based on their diagnosis, prior authorization is required (Rinehart-Thompson 2017d, 233).

74. **b** An audit trail is a record that shows who accessed a computer system, when it was accessed, and what operations were performed. These can be categorized as follows: individual accountability, reconstructing electronic events, problem monitoring, and intrusion detection (Sandefer 2016, 366).

75. **c** The Privacy Rule does not pre-empt or take precedence over the stricter or more stringent state statutes if the statutes provide individuals with greater privacy protections and give individuals greater rights with respect to their PHI (Biedermann and Dolezel 2017, 368).

76. **c** Spoliation is a legal concept applicable to both paper and electronic records. When evidence is destroyed that relates to a current or pending civil or criminal proceeding, it is reasonable to infer that the party had a guilty conscience or another motive to avoid the evidence (Klaver 2017a, 87–88).

77. **b** Reporting requirements mandate notification to the individual whose information was breached. In the case of breaches of more than 500 individuals' information, notification is also mandated to the media and the Secretary of Health and Human Services (Biedermann and Dolezel 2017, 401).

78. **a** Before an organization can decide on the methods for conducting the security risk analysis, they must consider their own characteristics and environment and implement reasonable and appropriate measures to protect against reasonably anticipated threats and hazards to the security of PHI. The security risk analysis process provides covered entities and business associates with the structural framework upon which to build their security plan (Biedermann and Dolezel 2017, 381).

79. **a** Addressable implementation specifications should be implemented unless an organization determines that the specification is not reasonable and appropriate. If this is the case then the organization must document why it is not reasonable and appropriate and adopt an equivalent measure if it is reasonable and appropriate to do so (Biedermann and Dolezel 2017, 380).

80. **b** When applying HIPAA, covered entities must also consider members of their workforce who may not be limited only to employees. The Privacy Rules defines workforce as employees, volunteers, trainees, and other persons whose conduct in the performance of work for a covered entity (CE) or business associate is under the direct control of such CE or business associate whether or not they are paid by the CE or business associate (Biedermann and Dolezel 2017, 354).

81. **b** Encryption is a technical method that reduces access and viewing of ePHI by unauthorized users. Encryption is defined as the process of transforming text into an unintelligible string of characters that can be transmitted via communications media with a high degree of security and then decrypted when it reaches a secure destination (AHIMA 2014, 55; Biedermann and Dolezel 2017, 394).

82. **a** The legal hold requires special, tracked handling of patient records to ensure no changes can be made in a record involved in litigation. This is common in the paper record environments to substantiate the integrity of the record and less common in the electronic environment where audit logs are the standard. Record managers need to address the use of legal hold for patient records in any information mode or medium (Biedermann and Dolezel 2017, 444–445).

83. **b** The Breach Notification Rule requires covered entities and business associates to establish policies and procedures to investigate an authorized use or disclosure of PHI to determine if a breach occurred, conclude the investigation, and to notify affected individuals and the Secretary of HHS within 60 days of date of discovery of the breach (Brinda and Watters 2016, 310–311).

84. **c** Expert Determination and Safe Harbor are Office of Civil Rights sanctioned HIPAA Privacy Rule deidentification methods. Deidentified information neither identifies nor provides a reasonable basis to identify an individual. There are two ways to deidentify information. (1) A formal determination is made by a qualified statistician. (2) The removal of specified identifiers of the individual and of the individual's relatives, household members, and employers is required, and is adequate only if the covered entity has no actual knowledge that the remaining information could be used to identify the individual (OCR 2012; Biedermann and Dolezel 2017, 359–361).

85. **c** The facility security plan should document the use of physical access controls. To meet the implementation specification, organizations should consider methods such as lock and key controls, security tagging equipment, using video cameras for surveillance, monitoring identification badges, and the use of human workforce to perform facilities security checks (Biedermann and Dolezel 2017, 391).

86. **d** The access control standard directs covered entities to implement technical policies and procedures for electronic information systems that maintain electronic protected health information in order to allow access only to those persons or software programs that have been granted access rights. Two required and two addressable implementation specifications are included in this standard. The two required specifications are the use of unique user identification and emergency access procedures. The two addressable specifications are automatic log off and encryption and decryption (Biedermann and Dolezel 2017, 394).

Domain 3

87. **d** A well-constructed RFP serves two important purposes. One is to solidify the planning information and organizational requirements into a single document, and the other is to provide valuable insights into the vendor's operations and products and to level the playing field in terms of asking all the vendors the same questions. This process requires skill and time (Amatayakul 2017, 198).

88. **b** Most organizations recognize that commercial products can meet their needs and that most of these products will far surpass the functionality that could be self-developed. Still, some organizations want to at least consider the build option. Some physicians are intrigued with developing their own perfect system, and some hospitals have development teams they do not want to give up. An organization's decision to build or buy should be based on a careful review of the marketplace. Currently, it is more expensive to undertake self-development. Unless self-development is coupled with a vendor partnership that leads to commercialization, a self-developed system can be a drawback when attempting to integrate with commercial products as the organization grows, merges, or acquires affiliates (Amatayakul 2017, 191).

89. **c** A table is an orderly arrangement of values that groups data into rows and columns. It should have specific, understandable headings for every column and row (Horton 2016, 249).

90. **c** The gross death rate is the proportion of all hospital discharges that ended in death. It is the basic indicator of mortality in a healthcare facility. The gross death rate is calculated by dividing the total number of deaths occurring in a given time period by the total number of discharges, including deaths, for the same time period: $25/500 = 0.05 \times 100 = 5\%$ (Palkie 2016b, 296).

91. **c** Running a mock query would be part of application testing that ensures every function of the new computer system works. Application testing also ensures the system meets the functional requirements and other required specifications in the RFP or contract (Sayles and Trawick 2014, 95).

92. **a** Bar charts are used to display data from one or more variables. The bars may be drawn vertically or horizontally. Bar charts are used for nominal or ordinal variables. In this case, you would be displaying the average length of stay by service and then within each service have a bar for each gender (Horton 2016, 257–258).

93. **c** Data warehouses are often hierarchical or multidimensional and are designed to receive very large volumes of data (often as an extraction of data from a repository) and perform complex, analytical processes on the data. Data can be mined and processed in many ways. For example, a data warehouse may be used for clinical quality improvement and best practice guideline development (Sandefer 2016, 376).

94. **b** A systematic random sample is a simple random sample that may be generated by selecting every fifth or every tenth member of the sampling frame. In order to ensure that a systematic random sample is truly random, the sample frame should not be sorted in an order that might bias the sample (White 2016a, 140).

95. **a** To achieve availability, an EHR must have full redundancy as well as backup and network redundancy. This means that there is a duplication of all data, hardware, cables, or other components of the system. Should the primary server crash, the system switches over to the second server and can continue processing (Sayles and Trawick 2014, 212).

96. **a** An indicator is a performance measure that enables healthcare organizations to monitor a process to determine whether it is meeting process requirements. Monitoring blood sugars on admission and discharge is an indicator of the quality of care delivered to the diabetes patient during the stay (Shaw and Carter 2015, 153).

97. **b** In data mining, the analyst performs exploratory data analysis to determine trends and identify patterns in the data set. Data mining is sometimes referred to as knowledge discovery. In healthcare, data mining may be used to determine if it is cost effective to expand facilities (White 2016b, 531).

98. **b** A pie chart is an easily understood chart in which the sizes of the slices of the pie show the proportional contribution of each part. Pie charts can be used to show the component parts of a single group or variable. In this case, the intent is to show the proportion of each payer to the whole payer mix (Marc 2016, 546).

99. **c** The incidence rate is a computation that compares the number of new cases of a specific disease for a given time period to the population at risk for the disease during the same time period (Oachs and Watters 2016, 1009).

100. **a** There is a discrepancy between the researcher's use of the term "anonymous" regarding informed consent and the researcher's intent to track respondents and nonrespondents. Anonymity demands that the researcher cannot link the response and the responder. The code would link the respondents to their data, so their data would no longer be anonymous (Klaver 2017c, 143–144).

101. **c** This type of data would be found on a dashboard report provided to the hospital's board of directors. The measures show a dramatic change in patient safety issues at this organization. The board would now need to investigate to determine why these changes occurred (Shaw and Carter 2015, 397).

102. **d** The patient meets the severity of illness with the vaginal bleeding but does not meet intensity of service because the surgery is not being performed as an inpatient. She would not meet the admission criteria provided (Shaw and Carter 2015, 147, 157).

103. **d** Organizational policy should address how personal health information provided by the patient will or will not be incorporated into the patient's health record. Copies of personal health records (PHR), created, owned, and managed by the patient are considered part of the legal health record when the organization uses them to provide treatment; however, the PHR does not replace the legal health record (Fahrenholz 2013a, 40).

104. **d** Surveys should be written at the reading level of the respondents, consistent formats should be used, all possible responses should be mutually exclusive, and terminology that the respondents understand should be incorporated. This survey used inconsistent formatting and did not have mutually exclusive responses in the age question (Shaw and Carter 2015, 132–134).

105. **c** Requirements analysis is the step that identifies, in detail, the precise requirements needed for both health information technology (that is, hardware and software) and operational components (people, policy, and process) of the health information system to meet the goals specified in the strategic plan (Amatayakul 2016, 400).

106. **b** The average length of stay (ALOS) is calculated from the total LOS. The total LOS divided by the number of patients discharged is the ALOS. Using the data provided, the ALOS for the 9 patients discharged on April 1 is 6 days (54/9) (Rossiter 2016, 495).

107. **a** Discrete data are whole numbers that may or may not be related, so a bar graph is the best data display tool to use (Shaw and Carter 2015, 80).

108. **a** In an application service provider (ASP) model, there is much less upfront capital outlay and fewer IT staff required in-house. In fact, the ASP acquisition strategy may be considered essentially a financing model (Amatayakul 2016, 402).

109. **c** Healthcare informatics is the field of information science concerned with the management of all aspects of health data and information through the application of computers and computer technologies (Oachs and Watters 2016, 1018).

110. **a** The opt-in model requires patients to specifically affirm their desire to have their data made available for exchange within an HIE. This option provides up-front control for patients since their data cannot be included unless they have agreed (Biedermann and Dolezel 2017, 306).

111. **d** Telehealth is "the use of electronic information and telecommunications technologies to support long-distance clinical healthcare, patient and professional health-related education, public health, and health administration (Sandefer 2016, 439).

112. **c** The weight of each MS-DRG is multiplied by the number of discharges for that MS-DRG to arrive at the total weight for each MS-DRG. The total weights are summed and divided by the number of total discharges to arrive at the case-mix index for a hospital. Calculation is as follows: $(0.9321 \times 10) + (0.7313 \times 20) + (1.4261 \times 10) + (0.9695 \times 20) + (0.7111 \times 10) = 64.709 / 70 = 0.9244$ (White 2016a, 155–156).

113. **a** In the analysis phase of the systems development life cycle (SDLC), it is important to examine the current system and identify opportunities for improvement or enhancement. Even though an initial assessment would be completed as part of the strategic information planning process, the analysis phase of the SDLC involves a more extensive evaluation (Amatayakul 2017, 46).

114. **c** The delivery of healthcare is increasingly complex; therefore, the related workflows are also increasingly complex. As the use of technology becomes critical in all aspects of patient care, understanding how the work flows within and between processes is critical. The success of information technology projects is not solely dependent on the technology, but also on the people and the process. Workflow analysis would uncover the human and process problems and should be done any time work involves multiple departments or functions and prior to identifying an information technology (IT) solution (Oachs 2016, 823).

115. **d** The HIE's record locator service (RLS) manages the pointers to the information on the servers of the HIE participants. The pointers in a RLS can include a person identification number (person ID) and metadata. The RLS does not provide information about the record, it merely points to where it might be found. Data are not stored in a centralized database and records are only provided when queried (McCann 2016, 454).

116. **b** Because of the number of tasks and their complexity and dependencies in EHR implementation, it is important to have an issues management program. An issues management program serves to receive and document issues and track them to their resolution (Amatayakul 2017, 258).

117. **b** Hospital Compare reports on 139 measures of hospital quality of care for heart attack, heart failure, pneumonia, and the prevention of surgical infections. The data available at Hospital Compare is reported by hospitals to meet the requirements of the Medicare Value Based Purchasing program. Hospitals that report all measures receive full payment updates from Medicare (White 2016a, 188).

118. **a** Duplicate health record numbers are when there is more than one unique identifier (for example, medical record number or person identifier) for the same person in the MPI. This causes one patient to have two or more different medical records within the same facility (Fahrenholz 2013c, 169).

119. **b** A review of the identified duplicates and overlays often reveals procedural problems that contribute to the creation of errors. Although health information management (HIM) departments may be the hub of identifying, mitigating, and correcting master patient index (MPI) errors, that information may never be shared with the registration department. If the registration staff is not aware of the errors, how can they begin to proactively prevent the errors from occurring in the first place? Registration process improvement activities can eventually reduce work for HIM departments. In addition, monitoring new duplicates is a critical process, and tracking reports should be created and implemented. Identifying and reporting MPI errors is important; however, tracking who made the error and why will decrease the number of duplicates (Fahrenholz 2013c, 171).

120. **c** Computer output laser disk/enterprise report management (COLD/ERM) technology electronically stores, manages, and distributes documents that are generated in a digital format and whose output data are report-formatted and print-stream originated. COLD/ERM technology not only electronically stores the report-formatted documents but also distributes them with fax, e-mail, web, and traditional hard copy print processes (Sandefer 2016a, 350).

121. **a** Application service providers (ASPs) are service firms that deliver, manage, and remotely host ("remote hosting" being a common term associated with ASPs) standardized (prepackaged) applications software through centralized servers via a network that are not exclusively but more commonly the Internet (Amatayakul 2016, 402).

122. **b** A pie chart is an easily understood chart in which the sizes of the slices of the pie show the proportional contribution of each part. Pie charts can be used to show the component parts of a single group or variable and are intended for interval or ratio data (Marc 2016, 546).

123. **a** A digital signature is a digitized version of a handwritten signature. A digitized signature differs from an electronic signature in that it uses handwritten signatures on a pen pad. The actual written signature is converted into an electronic image. Digitized signatures are acceptable if allowed by state, federal, and reimbursement regulations (Fahrenholz 2013b, 131).

124. **b** The employee turnover rate is over the internal benchmark for this hospital, so a performance improvement (PI) team should be formed to determine what the causes for this increase were. This increase in the turnover rate represents an opportunity for improvement (Shaw and Carter 2015, 29–30).

125. **c** The Joint Commission and CMS have identified several sets of core measures—sets of patient care characteristics that reflect the quality of care an organization can provide for important diagnoses. Pneumonia, congestive heart failure, and myocardial infarction are examples of current core measure sets that accredited organizations are required to collect data on. The summary reporting details how well the organization performed with respect to the measure in terms of percentage of compliance with the measures and shows how well the organization performed with respect to other similar organizations. HIV/AIDS and gastric ulcers are not among the current core measure sets (Shaw and Carter 2015, 169–170, 437).

126. **a** As the HIM department merges two duplicate records together, the source system (laboratory) also must be corrected. This creates new challenges for organizations because merge functionality could be different in each system or module, which in turn creates data redundancy. Addressing ongoing errors within the MPI means an established quality measurement and maintenance program is crucial to the future of healthcare (Fahrenholz 2013c, 171).

127. **c** Complete, publicly available standards are required to be able to exchange data and information effectively. The market needs to focus on interoperability, the ability of different systems to work seamlessly. In health information, interoperability is expected to include transmitting the meaning of data (Biedermann and Dolezel 2017, 302).

128. **d** Electronic data interchange (EDI) allows the transfer (incoming and outgoing) of information directly from one computer to another by using flexible, standard formats. This technology was first used in healthcare for the billing function (Sandefer 2016a, 354).

129. **b** When examining the correlation between two variables, the strength and direction of the relationship is measured. The next step in exploring the relationship between two variables is to analyze the ability of the value of one variable to predict an outcome or value of a second variable. In this scenario, the variable that is used to predict is called the independent variable (that is, age), and the outcome or variable to be predicted is called the dependent variable (that is, ancillary charges) (White 2016a, 122).

Domain 4

130. **c** Medical identity theft occurs when a patient uses another person's name and insurance information to receive healthcare benefits. Most often this is done so a person can receive medical care with an insurance benefit and pay less or nothing for the care he or she receives (Rinehart-Thompson 2016, 71).

131. **d** Upcoding is the practice of using a code that results in a higher payment to the provider that actually reflects the service or item provided (Hunt 2016, 286).

132. **a** Outpatient coding guidelines do not allow coding of possible conditions as a diagnosis for the patient. Do not code diagnoses documented as "probable," "suspected," "questionable," "rule out," "working diagnosis," or other similar terms indicating uncertainty. Rather, code the condition(s) to the highest degree of certainty for that encounter or visit, such as symptoms, signs, abnormal test results, or other reasons for the visit (Schraffenberger and Palkie 2017, 102).

133. **a** Clustering is the practice of coding or charging one or two middle levels of service codes exclusively under the philosophy that, although some will be higher and some lower, the charges will average out over an extended period (Kuehn 2017, 361).

134. **b** Licensure is the state's act of granting a healthcare organization or individual practitioner the right to provide healthcare services of a defined scope in a limited geographic area. State governments establish licensure requirements, which vary from state to state. Unlike accreditation, which is a voluntary process, licensure is mandatory. Licensure is required prior to a hospital's opening and providing medical services (Fahrenholz 2013b, 84).

135. **b** Capitated rate is a method of payment for health services in which the third-party payer reimburses providers a fixed, per capita amount for a period. *Per capita* means per head or per person. A common phrase in capitated contracts is per member per month (PMPM). The PMPM is the amount of money paid each month for each individual enrolled in the health insurance plan. Capitation is characteristic of HMOs (Casto and Forrestal 2015, 11).

136. **a** Home health agencies are expected to conduct an assessment that accurately reflects the patient's current health status and includes information to establish and monitor a plan of care. The plan of care must be reviewed and updated at least every 60 days or as often as the severity of the patient's condition requires (White 2013, 558).

137. **c** These procedures have been unbundled. Unbundling is the practice of coding services separately that should be coded together as a package because all the parts are included within one code and, therefore, one price. Unbundling done deliberately to obtain a higher reimbursement is a misrepresentation of services and can be considered fraud (Kuehn 2017, 361).

138. **d** Workers' compensation is a payer that pays for healthcare services due to work-related incidents. Because Workers' compensation is paying the bill, they are the third-party (Casto and Forrestal 2015, 8).

139. **c** A query may not be appropriate because the clinical information or clinical picture does not appear to support the documentation of a condition or procedure. In situations in which the provider's documented diagnosis does not appear to be supported by clinical findings, a healthcare entity's policies can provide guidance on a process for addressing the issue without querying the attending physician (Hunt 2016, 276–277).

140. **b** Episode-of-care reimbursement is a healthcare payment method in which providers receive one lump sum for all the services they provide related to a condition or disease (Casto and Forrestal 2015, 11).

141. **a** MS-DRG sets exist where the listings of diagnoses used to drive the grouping are the same. But, the presence or absence of a complication or comorbidity (CC) diagnosis or major complication or comorbidity (MCC) assigns the case to a higher or lower DRG. Undercoding can occur if coders fail to code as specific as possible and potentially miss CCs or MCCs (Casto and Forrestal 2015, 278).

142. **b** The explanation of benefits (EOB) is a report from a third-party payer that is sent from a healthcare insurer to the policy holder and provider. The EOB describes how the claim was processed by the healthcare insurer. It will include the actual charge for the service, the allowable amount under the payer agreement, the amount paid to the provider, and the remaining balance (if any) that the policy holder is obligated to pay (Casto and Forrestal 2015, 256).

143. **d** Recovery audit contractors work with a mission of reducing Medicare improper payments through detection and collection of overpayments, identification of underpayments, and implementation of actions that will prevent future improper payments (Casto and Forrestal 2015, 38).

144. **d** A notifiable disease is one for which regular, frequent, and timely information on individual cases is considered necessary to prevent and control disease. The list of notifiable diseases varies over time and by state; however, HIV/AIDS would be a notifiable disease anywhere (Edgerton 2016, 503–504).

145. **b** The quality of the documentation entered in the health record by providers can have major impacts on the ability of coding staff to perform their clinical analyses and assign accurate codes. In this situation, the best solution would be to educate the entire medical staff on their roles in the clinical documentation improvement process. Explaining to them the documentation guidelines and what documentation is needed in the record to support the more accurate coding of diabetes and its manifestations will reduce the need for coders to continue to query for this clarification (Hunt 2016, 275).

146. **c** Haldol is a drug frequently administered for behavior or mental conditions, so the coder would suspect mental or behavioral problems for this patient. The physician must be queried to confirm the diagnosis. Documentation is needed in the record to support the coding of the mental or behavioral problem (Hunt 2016, 276–277).

147. **b** As a result of the disparity in documentation practices by providers, querying has become a common communication and educational method to advocate proper documentation practices. Queries can be made in situations when there is clinical evidence for a higher degree of specificity or severity (Hunt 2016, 276–277).

148. **d** Integrated delivery system (IDS) is a term referring to the collaboration integration of healthcare providers. The goal of the IDS is a seamless delivery of care along the continuum of care, so one bill would be generated (Casto and Forrestal 2015, 109).

149. **d** The error rates are not comparable since there is no data about the number of records coded during the period by each coder. Work measurement is the process of studying the amount of work accomplished and the amount of work it takes to accomplish it. It involves the collection of data relevant to the work (Oachs 2016, 802).

150. **c** A claim scrubber is used by facilities as an internal auditing system to limit the number of denied claims (Casto and Forrestal 2015, 254).

151. **a** Fee-for-service reimbursement methodologies issue payments to healthcare providers on the basis of the charges assigned to each of the separate services that were performed for the patient. Chargemasters are used to list the individual charges for every element entailed in providing a service (for example, surgical supplies, surgical equipment, room and board, nursing care, respiratory therapy, pharmaceuticals, medical equipment, and so on) (Casto and Forrestal 2015, 9, 260).

152. **b** It is recommended that the healthcare entity's policy address the query format. A query generally includes the following information: patient name, admission date or date of service, health record number, account number, date query initiated, name and contact information of the individual initiating the query, and statement of the issue in the form of a question along with clinical indicators specified from the chart (for example, history and physical states urosepsis, lab reports WBC of 14,400, emergency department report fever of 102°F) (Hunt 2016, 279).

153. **a** The health information manager must continuously promote complete, accurate, and timely documentation to ensure appropriate coding, billing, and reimbursement. This requires a close working relationship with the medical staff, perhaps through the use of a physician advisor. Physician advisors assist in educating medical staff members on documentation needed for accurate billing. The medical staff is more likely to listen to a peer than to a facility employee, especially when the topic is documentation needed to ensure appropriate reimbursement (Hunt 2016, 275).

Domain 5

154. **b** The project champion is an executive in the organization who believes in the benefits of the project and advocates for the project. Depending on the overall impact the project has on the healthcare organization, this individual may be the manager of the HIM department or the director over the business unit where the HIM department resides, or it could be the chief operations officer (COO) (Olson 2016, 882).

155. **a** The external change agent has the advantage of providing a fresh, outside view as well as having the knowledge base to compare performance across organizations. Not having direct connections to the organization, he or she usually feels more comfortable challenging norms and culture, questioning unusual or unfair practices, and generally noting events that others may be reluctant to comment on. Being from the outside, he or she may be seen as having new skills and being more objective, or at least less biased, than an internal agent (Swenson 2016, 705).

156. **c** Many employers pay a slightly higher hourly wage to employees who work less desirable shifts (evening, night, weekend). This is referred to as shift differential (Oachs 2016, 794).

157. **d** First calculate the number of productive hours in a day: 88% × 8 hours = 7.04 hours/day. Then divide the 1,000 records/7 hours = 142.9 or 143 charts/hour for the three filers (Horton 2016, 185–187).

158. **c** The path with the greatest total duration time is called the critical path and represents the longest amount of time required to compete the total project. The critical path in this project is the sequence a → d → g → h → i, which will require 23 days (Shaw and Carter 2015, 454–455).

159. **d** Provisions of the FLSA, for example, cover minimum wage, overtime pay, child labor restrictions, and equal pay for equal work regardless of sex. Covered groups are referred to as nonexempt employees (LeBlanc 2016 ,725–726).

160. **c** Balanced scorecard methodology is a technique for measuring organization performance across the four perspectives of customer, financial, internal processes, and learning and growth (McClernon 2016, 951).

161. **c** An income statement summarizes the organization's revenue and expense transactions during the fiscal year. The income statement can be prepared at any point in time and reflects results up to that point (Revoir and Davis 2016, 849).

162. **b** The difference between the budgeted fees and actual fees is an unfavorable variance of $2,000. Unfavorable variances occur when the actual results are worse than what was budgeted (Revoir and Davis 2016, 862).

163. **d** American Health Information Management Association (AHIMA) professionals must abide to the AHIMA Code of Ethics principle to refuse to participate in or conceal unethical practices or procedures (Gordon and Gordon 2016, 915).

164. **b** To communicate effectively, managers must pay just as much attention to how their message is received and interpreted as they do to its content. In order to enhance the accuracy and acceptance of communication, the communicator needs to monitor others' nonverbal behaviors for cues that they are following or confused. Passive listening and distracted parties would not enhance effective communication (Kelly and Greenstone 2016, 36).

165. **d** Performance measurement is the process of comparing the outcomes of an organization, work unit, or employee to pre-established performance standards. The results of performance measurement are usually expressed as percentages, rates, ratios, averages, or other quantitative assessment. It is used to assess quality and productivity in clinical and administrative services. An 18 percent error rate on abstracting data is an indicator of a process problem in the health information management (HIM) department because it is an HIM function. The other items are not under the control of the HIM department and would not indicate a process problem in HIM (Oachs 2016, 803).

166. **b** In reengineering, the entire manner and purpose of a work process is questioned. The goal is to achieve the desired process outcome in the most effective and efficient manner possible. The results expected from reengineering efforts include increased productivity, decreased costs, improved quality, maximized revenue, and more satisfied customers. However, it should be clearly understood that the main focus is on reducing costs (Oachs 2016, 819).

167. **b** Strategic thinking is a way of introducing innovation into decision making and engaging others in the process of change. The skills that distinguish a strategic thinker include the ability to plan and strategize, flexibility and creativity, comfort with uncertainty and risk, a sense of urgency and vision of how to move change forward positively, being able to gain a powerful core of organizational supporters and customers, and the capability to communicate the vision and plans (McClernon 2016, 929).

168. **b** Mentoring is a form of coaching. A mentor is a senior employee who works with employees early in their careers, giving them advice on developing skills and career options (Patena 2016, 761).

169. **c** After employees have been recruited and selected, the first step is to introduce them to the organization and their immediate work setting and functions. New employee orientation includes a group of activities that introduce the employee to the organization's mission, policies, rules, and culture; the department or workgroup; and the specific job he or she will be performing (Patena 2016, 756).

170. **c** Conceptual skills, especially at the higher levels of the organization, include such competencies as visioning the organization, planning, decision making, problem solving, creativity, and conceptualizing the connections among parts of a complex organizational system or "systems thinking" (Swenson 2016, 681).

171. **b** Every project has an identified sponsor. The sponsor is the facility employee with the most vested interest in the project's success. It is a good practice to select someone who has responsibility for the organization's departments, divisions, and personnel that will be affected by the project (Olson 2016, 881).

172. **c** The current ratio compares total current assets with total current liabilities:

$$\frac{4{,}000{,}000}{5{,}000{,}000}=\frac{4}{5}=0.8$$

$$\frac{\text{Total current assets}}{\text{Total current liabilities}}$$

From this information, one can take the current assets (cash + accounts receivable + inventory) divided by current liabilities (accounts payable) to arrive at current ratio. The current ratio indicates that for every dollar of current liability, $0.80 of current assets could be used to discharge the liability, which is not enough because it is not at least $1 (Revoir and Davis 2016, 852).

173. **d** In this case, a profitability index helps the organization prioritize investment opportunities. For each investment, divide the present value of the cash inflows by the present value of the cash outflows. The profitability index for each investment is calculated in the figure below. Each investment is equally profitable, as all three have the same profitability index of 4 (Revoir and Davis 2016, 868).

	Radiology	Cardiology	Pharmacy
Present value of cash inflows	$2,000,000	$1,200,000	$40,000
Present value of cash outflows	$500,000	$300,000	$10,000
Profitability Index	$2,000,000/$500,000 = 4	$1,200,000/$300,000 = 4	$40,000/$10,000 = 4

174. **d** Internal change agents have the clear advantage of being familiar with the organization, its history, subtle dynamics, secrets, and resources. Such people are often well respected, securely positioned, and have the strong interpersonal relationships to foster change. There is an advantage to recognizing the internal expertise of employees, maintaining confidentiality of the process, and using people who are invested in the success of the outcome (Swenson 2016, 705).

175. **a** Qualitative standards specify the level of service from a function such as accuracy rate, error rate, turnaround time, and response time In this case, timely response to release of information requests can indirectly impact patient care. To properly communicate performance standards, managers need to make the distinction between quantitative and qualitative standards and identify examples of each for the health information systems (HIS) functions (Oachs 2016, 799–800).

176. **b** A Gantt chart is used to illustrate project tasks, phases, and milestones and their start, end, and completion dates. It helps to illustrate where more than one task must be performed simultaneously. The column labeled as B shows a check mark indicating the task "Load test data" is completed (Amatayakul 2017, 243).

177. **c** One thing that binds team members together is having a common purpose. The purpose for an ongoing work team, for example, might be to ensure cross-training, improve procedures, and monitor quality and productivity. A common purpose is necessary in order to achieve team building (LeBlanc 2016, 738).

178. **a** When a manager is planning to contract for staffing in a transitional situation in order to meet organizational goals, various types of arrangements can be considered. Full-service contracting would be handing off a complete function to the contracted company (Oachs 2016, 797).

179. **b** In-service education is a continuous process that builds on the basic skills learned through new employee orientation and on-the-job training. In-service education is concerned with teaching employees specific skills and behaviors required to maintain job performance or to retrain workers whose jobs have changed (Patena 2016, 762).

180. **a** The strong matrix organization is very similar to the balanced matrix but includes a department of project managers. In these organizations, project managers are not functional staff members assuming the role of project manager but rather project manager specialists reporting to a manager of project management. The strong matrix organizations provide the project manager a moderate to high level of authority over the project and project resources (Olson 2016, 885).

Exam 2 Answers

Domain 1

1. **a** The purpose of the Data Elements for Emergency Department Systems (DEEDS) is to support the uniform collection of data in hospital-based emergency departments and to substantially reduce incompatibilities in emergency department records. DEEDS contains recommendations on both the content and structure of the data elements to be collected (Giannangelo 2015, 254).

2. **c** Health records and other documentation related to patient care are the property of the hospital or healthcare provider that created them. However, the information in each record belongs to the individual patient (Fahrenholz 2013a, 26).

3. **c** Precision often relates to numerical data. It denotes how close to an actual size, weight, or other standard a particular measurement is (Sharp and Madlock-Brown 2016, 197).

4. **c** Applicable statutes of limitations, the time period in which a lawsuit may be filed, must be considered in establishing a retention schedule (Rinehart-Thompson 2017c, 195).

5. **c** The operative report should be written or dictated immediately after surgery and filed in the patient's health record as soon as possible. Some hospitals may require surgeons to include brief descriptions of the operations in their postoperative progress notes when delays in dictation or transcription are unavoidable. Other caregivers can then refer to the progress note until the final operative report becomes available (Russo 2013a, 256).

6. **a** A consultation report is the documented findings or recommendation for further treatment by a physician or specialist. Consultations are usually performed at the request of the attending physician (Russo 2013a, 215).

7. **d** A discharge summary must be completed within 30 days after discharge for most patients but within 24 hours for patients transferred to other facilities. Discharge summaries are not always required for patients who were hospitalized for less than 48 hours (Reynolds and Sharp 2016, 115).

8. **b** The destruction of patient-identifiable clinical documentation should be carried in accordance with relevant federal and state regulations as well as organizational policy. Health records related to open investigations, audits, or court cases should not be destroyed for any reason. Paper-based health records can be destroyed using any of the following methods: burning, shredding, pulping, or pulverizing (Fahrenholz 2013b, 111).

9. **a** Data governance is an iterative process. It initially prioritizes initiatives and focuses on small select business imperatives that quickly deliver value and expand as the program matures (Johns 2016, 88).

10. **c** A longitudinal health record maintains information throughout the lifespan of the patient, ideally from birth to death (Fahrenholz 2013a, 45).

11. **a** The physician principally responsible for the patient's hospital care generally dictates the discharge summary. However, a resident, physician assistant, or nurse practitioner who is being supervised by the attending physician may complete this task. Regardless of who documents it, the attending physician is responsible for the content and quality of the summary and must date and sign it (Russo 2013a, 284).

12. **d** An interval note may be used for the patient's history and physical when the patient is readmitted within 30 days of the initial treatment for the same condition (Russo 2013a, 207).

13. **d** The principal procedure is the procedure that was performed for the definitive treatment (rather than the diagnosis) of the main condition or a complication of the condition (Schraffenberger and Palkie 2017, 83).

14. **b** An HIM professional must be aware of the retention statutes and retention periods in his or her state of employment and any federal statutes that apply. In some cases, the organization may define a retention period that is longer than the period required by the state. The organization should base its retention policy on hospital and medical needs and any applicable statutes and regulations (Reynolds and Sharp 2016, 133).

15. **b** A pathology report is a document that contains the diagnosis determined by examining cells and tissues under a microscope. The report may also contain information about the size, shape, and appearance of a specimen as it looks to the naked eye. This information is known as the gross description (Russo 2013a, 256, 259).

16. **d** A vocabulary standard is a common definition for medical terms to encourage consistent descriptions of an individual's condition in the health record (Sayles and Trawick 2014, 170–171).

17. **b** The results of the inventory indicate a significant problem and should not be ignored. Before in-service training or memos can be developed, the organization's formal position on data dictionaries must be established through development of a policy and associated standards. An organization-wide data dictionary is developed outside the framework of a specific database design process. This data dictionary serves to promote data quality through data consistency across the organization. Individual data element definitions are agreed upon and defined. This leads to better quality data and facilitates the detailed, technical data dictionaries that are integrated with the databases themselves (Sharp and Madlock-Brown 2016, 198).

18. **a** This model shows that the relationship between the data table (or entity) HOSPITAL and the data table (or entity) DIVISION is one-to-many. A one-to-many relationship means that for every instance of HOSPITAL stored in the database, many related instances of DIVISION may be stored. Reading the diagram in the other direction, each instance of DIVISION stored in the database is related to only one instance of HOSPITAL (Sayles and Trawick 2014, 56).

19. **a** Migration of data of all kinds needs to be established as systems are established and changed. Standards-based technology is essential to continued operational efficiency and integrity of older, but still useful, data and documents. Some hospitals talk about having an electronic medical record (EMR) because all paper is now electronic due to the document imaging system. Such a system supports improved access to information and this is part of the migration path (Biedermann and Dolezel 2017, 444).

20. **a** The patient has esophageal reflux with no esophagitis mentioned, therefore K21.9 is the correct diagnosis code. For the ICD-10-PCS procedure code, a closed biopsy of the esophagus was performed via esophagoscopy and therefore 0DB58ZX is the correct code. The Section is Medical and Surgical—character 0; Body System is Gastrointestinal—character D; Root Operation is Excision—character B; Body Part is Esophagus—character 5; Approach—Via a Natural or Artificial Opening Endoscopic—character 8; No Device—character Z; and the procedure was for diagnostic reasons—character X (Schraffenberger and Palkie 2017, 34; Kuehn and Jorwic, 2017, 21–23, 77).

21. **d** One disadvantage of paper-based health records is the inability of an access control mechanism. Controlling access is an important aspect of maintaining the legal integrity of the record. In the paper world, this is controlled through physical security safeguards, chart tracking, and outguide systems (Fahrenholz and Russo 2013, 145).

22. **a** An accession number consists of the first digits of the year the patient was first seen at the facility, with the remaining digits assigned sequentially throughout the year. The first case in, for example, might be 09-0001. The accession number may be assigned manually or by the automated cancer database used by the organization. An accession registry of all cases can be kept manually or be provided as a report by the database software (Sharp and Madlock-Brown 2016, 174).

23. **d** Each progress note should include changes in the patient's condition, findings based on the facts of the case, test results and response to treatment, as well as an analysis of the findings. The final part of the note contains the decisions or actions planned for future care. Flowcharts are another effective way to illustrate the patient's progress and can be computerized to demonstrate progress or to keep track of certain data. The patient's condition dictates how often progress notes are recorded, and the frequency is generally established by the healthcare facility or payers of care. In a hospital, the physician primarily responsible for the patient's care is often required to write a progress note daily. Charting by exception would not be an acceptable method to record patient progress notes (Reynolds and Sharp 2016, 111, 112).

24. **b** The primary key (PK) for PATIENT, PATIENT_MRN, is repeated in VISIT, as is the PK for CLINIC, CLINIC_ID. These keys are called foreign keys (FK) in the VISIT table. Foreign keys allow relationships between tables. By having the foreign keys in VISIT, the information in PATIENT and CLINIC is linked through the VISIT table (Johns 2015, 127–128).

25. **c** Reliability is a measure of consistency of data items based on their reproducibility and an estimation of their error of measurement (Sharp and Madlock-Brown 2016, 197).

26. **c** Medicare Conditions of Participation require that admitting physicians perform an initial physical examination within 24 hours of admission. Documentation of medical history, consents, and the physical examination must be available in the patient's record before any surgical procedures can be performed (Russo 2013a, 207).

27. **b** Main term: Depression, subterm: recurrent; see Disorder, depressive, recurrent. Follow the cross reference to Disorder, depressive, recurrent, severe F33.2 (Schraffenberger and Palkie 2017, 34).

28. **c** The Excludes1 note indicates that the conditions listed after it cannot ever be used at the same time as the code above the Excludes1 note. The conditions listed in the code and in the Excludes1 note are mutually exclusive. A patient cannot have both conditions at the same time (Schraffenberger and Palkie 2017, 18).

29. **a** In peer review, a member of a profession assesses the work of colleagues within that same profession. Peer review has traditionally been at the center of quality assessment and assurance efforts. The medical profession's peer review efforts have emphasized the scientific aspects of quality. Appropriate use of pharmaceuticals, postoperative infection rates, and accuracy of diagnosis are among the measures of quality that have been used. Peer review is a requirement of both CMS and the Joint Commission (Fuller 2016, 29).

30. **a** Because of the risks associated with miscommunication, verbal orders are strongly discouraged. To reduce miscommunication, the person receiving the order should read it back to ensure the order is correct. Verbal orders should be authenticated as soon as possible after they are given (Rinehart-Thompson 2017c, 178–179).

31. **c** Begin with the main term of hernia repair; inguinal; incarcerated. The age of the patient and the fact that the hernia is not recurrent make the choice 49507 (Kuehn 2017, 22–24, 168–170).

32. **d** An entity becomes a table in your relational database because it is the person, place, or thing about which you are collecting the data in your database. You would need to be able to query data on each entity from the database (White 2016a, 46).

33. **c** Hospitals and other healthcare facilities develop health record retention polices to ensure that health records comply with all applicable state and federal regulations and accreditation standards and meet future patient-care needs. Retention policies dictate how long individual health records must remain available for authorized use (Fahrenholz 2013b, 109–110).

34. **b** Structured data can have many benefits include completeness, quality, and accessibility of the data for a variety of purposes. Structured data are often entirely appropriate and highly recommended for data entry when the options are limited or are required to conform to a specific standard (Biedermann and Dolezel 2017, 159).

35. **b** A database is a term used to refer to an organized collection of data that have been stored electronically to facilitate easy access (Russo 2013b, 322).

36. **b** Most health record systems are organized according to one of two database models—the centralized or distributed—or a hybrid of the two models. In the centralized database model, all of the organization's patient health information is stored in one system (Russo 2013b, 322).

37. **a** Continuity of care record (CCR) is documentation of care delivery from one healthcare experience to another (Palkie 2016a, 162).

38. **a** Although registries and databases are almost universally computerized, data collection is sometimes done manually. The most frequent method is abstracting, the process of reviewing the patient health records and entering the required data elements into the database (Sharp and Madlock-Brown 2016, 191).

39. **c** Occlusion is the correct root operation. An occlusion procedure has the objective of complete closure and can involve a natural or artificial opening for procedures on the orifices. In this scenario, the blood supply to the malignant tumor is completely closed off to prevent growth (Kuehn and Jorwic 2017, 116).

40. **a** The Healthcare Effectiveness Data and Information Set (HEDIS) is a set of standard performance measures designed to provide purchasers and consumers of healthcare with the information they need for comparing the performance of managed healthcare plans (Shaw and Carter 2015, 179).

41. **a** Data quality management functions involve continuous improvement for data quality throughout an organization and include four key processes for data. These processes are application, collection, warehousing, and analysis. Analysis is the process of translating data into information utilized for an application (White 2013b, 554).

Domain 2

42. **b** Only when copies of the personal health record (PHR) are used for treatment can they be considered part of the facilities' legal health record; however, the PHR does not replace the legal health record (Fahrenholz 2013a, 40).

43. **c** Context-based access is the most stringent type of access control. It takes into account the person attempting to access the data, the type of data being accessed, and the context of the transaction in which the access attempt is made (Sayles and Trawick 2014, 220).

44. **d** Risk analysis is a systematic process of identifying security measures to afford protections given an organization's specific environment, including where the measures are located, what level of automation they have, how sensitive the information is that needs protection, what remediation will cost, and many other factors (Brinda and Watters 2016, 320).

45. **b** As within any type of setting, a common security threat to a health information system is an internal threat within the organization by employees (Amatayakul 2017, 371–372).

46. **b** The basic elements of an informed consent should include the purpose of the proposed procedure, any risks associated with the procedure, and if any noninvasive treatment alternatives are available (Klaver 2017c, 141).

47. **b** Entity authentication is the verification of a user's identity. Simply put, this standard seeks to ensure that organizations put methods in place to verify that users are who they claim they are (Biedermann and Dolezel 2017, 395).

48. **c** Firewalls are hardware and software security devices situated between the routers of a private and public network. They are designed to protect computer networks from unauthorized outsiders. However, they also can be used to protect entities within a single network, for example, to block laboratory technicians from getting into payroll records. Without firewalls, IT departments would have to deploy multiple-enterprise security programs that would soon become difficult to manage and maintain (Sandefer 2016a, 366).

49. **d** A regulation is a rule established by an administrative agency of government (Rinehart-Thompson 2016, 45).

50. **c** Vulnerability is defined as an inherent weakness or absence of a safeguard that could be exploited by a threat. Vulnerabilities are grouped into either technical or nontechnical categories with technical vulnerabilities reflecting inappropriate information systems protective methods. Nontechnical vulnerabilities are demonstrated by such things as policy and procedure weaknesses (Biedermann and Dolezel 2017, 381).

51. **b** The security audit process should include triggers that identify the need for a closer inspection. Just because a trigger has been activated does not mean that there has been a breach. With common names such as Smith and Jones, it would be easy for an employee named Smith or Jones to access patient information for an unrelated person with the same last name (Sayles and Trawick 2014, 215–216).

52. **b** The identification of and response to security incidents (or events) is the required implementation specification. Response and reporting is the single required implementation specification that states covered entities must identify and respond to suspected or known security incidents; mitigate, to the extent practicable, harmful events of security incidents that are known to the covered entity; and document security incidents and their outcomes (Biedermann and Dolezel 2017, 387).

53. **c** Granting clinical privileges refers to the authorizing of a practitioner to provide specific patient care services within well-defined limits. The criteria for awarding clinical privileges must be detailed in the medical staff bylaws or rules and regulations (Fuller 2016, 16).

54. **d** The distinction of psychotherapy notes is important due to HIPAA requirements that these notes may not be released unless specifically identified in an authorization (Munn 2013, 616–617).

55. **c** The Omnibus Rule created a new fine structure for civil monetary penalties based on a four-tier system for HIPAA violations. Tiers 3 and 4 are based on violations that have been determined to be due to willful neglect. In this situation, because the breach was corrected within 30 days from the date of discovery it would fall into Tier 3. If it wasn't corrected, it would be a Tier 4 violation (Brinda and Watters 2016, 311–132).

56. **c** The Privacy Rule's general requirement is that authorization must be obtained for uses and disclosure of protected health information (PHI) created for research that includes treatment of the individual (Rinehart-Thompson 2017d, 225).

57. **d** The Patient Self-Determination Act, which is part of the Omnibus Budget Reconciliation Act of 1990, requires healthcare providers to inform patients of their right to create advance directives, document the presence or absence of an advance directive in a patient's health record, and ensure compliance with state law respecting advance directives (Klaver 2017c, 151–152).

58. **c** Allowing employees of a covered entity to access their own protected health information electronically results in a situation in which the covered entity may be in compliance with parts of the HIPAA Privacy Rule, but in violation of other sections of the Privacy Rule. An ideal situation would be to establish a patient portal through which all patients may view their own records in a secure manner, and for which an employee has neither more or less rights than any other patient (Thomason 2013, 109).

59. **b** By virtue of their age, minors are generally considered legally incompetent and unable to consent to their own treatment. Therefore, the consent of a parent or other legal guardian is required. If the minor's parents are divorced, only one parent needs to consent for treatment (Klaver 2017c, 160).

60. **d** The Security Risk Analysis process provides covered entities (CEs) and business associates (BAs) with the structural framework upon which to build their HIPAA Security Plan. The value of a risk analysis stems from its uniqueness to the specific organization in which it is conducted. Every organization is different and every risk analysis should reflect the unique and complex interrelationships between a multitude of systems, processes, and policies that in combination result in that specific organization's HIPAA Security Plan (Biedermann and Dolezel 2017, 381).

61. **a** The information access management standard is focused on policies and procedures that, based upon the entity's access authorization policies, establish, document, review, and modify a user's right of access to a workstation, transaction, program, or process (Biedermann and Dolezel 2017, 386).

62. **d** A strategy included in a good security program is an employee security awareness program. Employees are often responsible for threats to data security. Consequently, employee awareness is a particularly important tool in reducing security breaches (Reynolds and Brodnik 2017a, 274).

63. **d** Redisclosure is the process of releasing health record documentation originally created by a different provider. Federal and state regulations provide specific redisclosure guidelines. When in doubt, follow the same release and disclosure guidelines for other types of health information (AHIMA 2009; Fahrenholz 2013, 104).

64. **c** The Privacy Rule introduced the standard that individuals should be informed of how covered entities use or disclose protected health information (PHI). This notice must be provided to an individual at his or her first contact with the covered entity (Rinehart-Thompson 2017d, 219).

65. **a** There are circumstances in which PHI can be used or disclosed without the individual's written authorization and for which the individual does not have the opportunity to agree or object. These would include use and disclosure of medical information for treatment, payment, and operations. Utilization review is use of the information for operations. Sending records to a physician for continuity of care would be for treatment purposes (Rinehart-Thompson 2017d, 225–226).

66. **b** The Privacy Rule lists two circumstances where protected health information (PHI) can be used or disclosed without the individual's authorization (although the individual must be informed in advance and given an opportunity to agree or object). One of these circumstances is disclosing PHI to a family member or a close friend that is directly relevant to his or her involvement with the patient's care or payment. Likewise, a covered entity may disclose PHI, including the patient's location, general condition, or death, to notify or assist in the notification of a family member, personal representative, or some other person responsible for the patient's care (Rinehart-Thompson 2017d, 225–226).

67. **c** The custodian of health records is the individual who has been designated as having responsibility for the care, custody, control, and proper safekeeping and disclosure of health records for such persons or institutions that prepare and maintain records of healthcare (Brodnik 2017a, 9).

68. **c** Competent adults have a general right to consent to or refuse medical treatment. If an adult has a sound mind or did when he or she created a living will, this patient has the right to refuse treatment (Klaver 2017c, 154–155).

69. **b** The law firm of Hall and Hall is a business associate of Champion Hospital because it performs activities on behalf of the hospital and uses and discloses individually identifiable information. A business associate is a person or organization other than a member of a covered entity's workforce that performs functions or activities on behalf of or affecting a covered entity that involve the use or disclosure of individually identifiable health information (45 CFR 160.103(1); Rinehart-Thompson 2017d, 211).

70. **b** Facility access controls include establishing safeguards to prohibit the physical hardware and computer system itself from unauthorized access while ensuring that proper authorized access is allowed (Reynolds and Brodnik 2017a, 275–276).

71. **c** Audit trails are used to facilitate the determination of security violations and to identify areas for improvement. In this case, the audit trail review should be used to begin an investigation into what exactly the employee printed and why (Brinda and Watters 2016, 366–367).

72. **b** In the HIPAA Security Rule, one of the technical safeguards standards is access control. This includes automatic log-off, which ensures electronics processes that terminate an electronic session after a predetermined time of inactivity (Reynolds and Brodnik 2017a, 277).

73. **c** When obtaining consent for treatment, the physician is the healthcare provider who would discuss the treatment with the patient. The basic elements of an informed consent should include the purpose of the proposed procedure, any risks associated with the procedure, and if any noninvasive treatment alternatives are available (Klaver 2017c, 141).

74. **c** Covered entities (CEs) are responsible for their workforce, which consists not only of employees but also volunteers, student interns, and trainees. Workforce members are not limited to those who receive wages from the CE (45 CFR 160.103(1); Rinehart-Thompson 2017d, 211).

75. **b** Although a person or organization may, by definition, be subject to the Privacy Rule by virtue of the type of organization it is, not all information that it holds or comes into contact with is protected by the Privacy Rule. For example, the Privacy Rule has specifically excluded from its scope employment records held by the covered entity in its role as employer (45 CFR 160.103). Under this exclusion, employee physical examination reports contained within personnel files are specifically exempted from this rule (Rinehart-Thompson 2017d, 215).

76. **c** Contingency or disaster recovery planning (DRP) is an important component of protecting ePHI. Healthcare providers need plans in the event of a power failure, disaster, or other emergency that limits or eliminates access to facilities and ePHI (Brinda and Watters 2016, 322).

77. **c** Shared coding in information systems can include the use of standard identifiers. The original HIPAA legislation required adoption of four identifiers: employers, providers, health plans, and individuals. Three were implemented: the Employer Identification Number (EIN), the National Provider Identifier (NPI), and the Health Plan Identifier (HPID). The unique healthcare identifier for individuals has been put on hold (Amatayakul 2017, 411–412).

78. **b** The Privacy Rule permits individuals to request that a covered entity amend a PHI or a record about the individual in a designated record set. Because the incident report was erroneously placed in this patient's record, it is not part of the designated record set and not amendable by the patient (Rinehart-Thompson 2017e, 246–247).

79. **c** The HIPAA Privacy Rule concept of "minimum necessary" does not apply to disclosures made for treatment purposes. However, the covered entity must define, within the organization, what information physicians need as part of their treatment role (Rinehart-Thompson 2017d, 234).

80. **c** Determination if a breach has occurred should be completed before action is taken. The audit trail is a software program that tracks every single access to data in the computer system. It logs the name of the individual who accessed the data, the date and time, and the action taken (for example, modifying, reading, or deleting data). Depending on the organization's policy, audit trails are reviewed periodically or on predetermined schedules. Audit trails document when data have been accessed and by whom. Review of audit trails can help detect whether a breach of security has occurred (Rinehart-Thompson 2017e, 250–251).

81. **b** Covered entities (CEs) must respond to requests to access PHI within 30 days. There can be a further 30-day extension however, but the first response must be within 30 days (Rinehart-Thompson 2017e, 245).

82. **c** The 2013 HIPAA Omnibus Rule finalized regulations give patients the right to request that their PHI not be disclosed to a health plan if they pay out of pocket in full for the services or items. A provider who accepts the payment and provides the service is compelled to abide by this request (Rinehart-Thompson 2017d, 220–221).

83. **b** The review of the health record by a medical staff committee is approved use of protected health information (PHI). The Privacy Rule provides a broad list of activities that fall under the umbrella of healthcare operations including quality assessment and improvement and case management (Rinehart-Thompson 2017d, 216–217).

84. **b** An EHR system can afford better security for PHI because authentication systems, access controls, audit logs, and other measures exist which are not possible in a paper environment (Fahrenholz 2013b, 145).

85. **c** The process of disclosing health record documentation originally created by a different provider is called redisclosure. In the interest of patient care, health records from other facilities should be made part of the designated record set at the current facility if that information is needed for diagnosis or treatment, and if state law does not otherwise prohibit it (Rinehart-Thompson 2017d, 231–232).

86. **c** Given that a unit level password could be used by any worker on a unit, it does not verify that a person is who they claim to be. The Person or Entity Authentication Standard seeks to ensure that organizations put methods in place to verify that users are who they claim they are. Passwords, smart cards, tokens, fobs, and biometrics are some of the many methods used in healthcare settings to confirm user identity (Biedermann and Dolezel 2017, 395).

Domain 3

87. **c** In data mining, the analyst performs exploratory data analysis to determine trends and identify patterns in the data set (White 2016b, 531).

88. **a** Monitoring and managing a master patient index (MPI) also requires constant vigilance from the organization, including oversight, evaluation, and correction of errors. The overall responsibility of maintaining the MPI should be centralized and given to an individual who is detail oriented, is properly trained, has access to adequate tools, and is well versed in the organization's policies and procedures for MPI maintenance. Working with the organization's integration team to ensure ADT interfaces are properly built and tested is a key responsibility of the MPI manager (Reynolds and Sharp 2016, 130).

89. **b** It is critical that the organization's information system (IS) plans be well aligned and integrated with its overall organizational strategic plans. To develop a tactical plan for IS technology, the healthcare organization should engage in strategic IS planning (Amatayakul 2016, 389).

90. **c** Data are the raw elements that make up our communications. Humans have the innate ability to combine data they collect and, through all their senses, produce information (which is data that have been combined to produce value) and enhance that information with experience and trial-and-errors that produce knowledge. In this example, the gender is tied to race in the data collection that constitutes information and not a data element (Amatayakul 2017, 284).

91. **d** Data are the raw elements that make up our communications. Humans have the innate ability to combine data they collect and, through all their senses, produce information (which is data that have been combined to produce value) and enhance that information with experience and trial-and-errors that produce knowledge. The average length of stay is specific to 5.6 days at Holt Hospital. This is meaningful information because it is a statistic for a specific location. The other distractors are merely data as they have no context (Amatayakul 2017, 284).

92. **c** The patient portal allows a patient to access all or part of the health record that is maintained by the patient's provider (Amatayakul 2017, 15).

93. **c** The normal distribution is actually a theoretical family of distributions that may have any mean or any standard deviation. It is bell-shaped and symmetrical about the mean. Because it is symmetrical, 50 percent of the observations fall above the mean and 50 percent fall below it. In a normal distribution, the mean, median, and mode are equal (White 2016b, 523).

94. **c** Clinical decision support systems automatically analyze health record data and search for unusual patterns. When it identifies a potential problem (for example, a drug interaction or drug allergy), the system issues an alert or a reminder that includes a recommendation for specific corrected action (Russo 2013b, 326).

95. **c** A line graph or plot is used to display time trends. The x-axis shows the unit of time from left to right, and the y-axis measures the number of prostate cancer deaths (Marc 2016, 546).

96. **d** Researchers use convenience samples when they "conveniently" use any unit that is at hand. For example, HIM professionals investigating physician satisfaction with departmental services could interview physicians who came to the department (Forrestal 2016, 593).

97. **a** These data are showing that Doctor X bills code 99213 primarily and not the other four service codes for established patients. However, the graph tells the reader nothing about Doctor X's documentation which would make answers b and c incorrect. Doctor X does use 99212 less than his peers, not more than his peers. A physician who consistently reports the same level of service for all patient encounters may look suspicious to claims auditors. With the exception of certain specialists, physicians treat all types of patients in their offices, and office treatment requires use of most of the levels of services (Kuehn 2017, 41–42).

98. **d** The MPI includes data elements necessary to identify a patient. These elements include date of birth, complete address, phone numbers, health record number, billing or account number, name of attending physician, dates of admission and discharge, disposition, marital status, gender, race, and patient's emergency contact (Reynolds 2016, 130).

99. **b** The patient meets severity of illness with the persistent fever and intensity of service with the inpatient-approved surgery scheduled within 24 hours of admission (Shaw and Carter 2015, 147, 157).

100. **d** A line graph or plot may be used to display time trends. The x-axis shows the unit of time from left to right, and the y-axis measures the values of the variable being plotted (Marc 2016, 546).

101. **a** Whether the master patient index (MPI) is at a local, enterprise, or HIE level, its primary purpose is to facilitate the link between clinical and administrative information between disparate systems. With so many patient care and industry initiatives at stake, the quality of MPI data can no longer be considered a back-end function. Errors in MPI databases can lead to billing problems, unnecessary duplicate tests, and potential legal exposure. In addition, duplicates contribute to HIM operational workload and create inefficiencies as each new patient receives a new medical record number, file folder (in the paper world), and staff time in MPI maintenance activities (Fahrenholz 2013c, 171).

102. **a** Due diligence can be in the form of site visits, corporate visits, reference checks, credit checks on owners of the vendor company, and other steps needing to be performed before a final contract is negotiated to ensure that the organization is getting the product it wants (Amatayakul 2016, 403–404).

103. **d** In this situation there are too many changes occurring at the same time to determine what is improving the nursing staffing satisfaction scores. Any one item could be the reason for the improvement. To evaluate the impact of the electronic health record (EHR) nursing documentation component, a benefits realization study should have been utilized. This would have studied the impact of the EHR component before and after implementation (Amatayakul 2017, 106).

104. **a** The graph shows that the Asian population has increased in the last five years, so the organization may need to adjust staffing, offer a wider variety in dietary choices, and ensure patient rights and safety are appropriate in the face of possible language barriers and cultural differences (Shaw and Carter 2015, 95–97).

105. **d** A gross autopsy rate is the proportion or percentage of deaths that are followed by the performance of autopsy. Using this data, five patients had autopsies performed out of the 25 deaths; therefore, 5/25 = 0.2 × 100 = 20% (Edgerton 2016, 498).

106. **b** Interoperability is often described in levels. The NCVHS has identified three levels: basic, functional, and semantic. Basic interoperability relates to the ability to successfully transmit and receive data from one computer to another. Functional interoperability refers to sending messages between computers with a shared understanding of the structure and format of the message. The use of clinical terminologies in EHRs to provide standardized data is essential to achieving semantic interoperability (Palkie 2016a, 153).

107. **c** The mode is used to indicate the most frequent observation in a frequency distribution. In this data set there are three occurrences of the value 8 and only two or less occurrences of any other value, so 8 is the mode (Edgerton 2016, 486).

108. **c** Sampling is used when examining the entire population is either too time consuming or too expensive. A sample is the subset of the population or universe. The universe is the set of all units that are eligible to be sampled. A listing of all of the subjects in the universe is called the sampling frame. The universe in a sampling plan may be patients, physicians, health records, or any other unit of analysis that is studied. In this case the sample unit is the claim (White 2016a, 135).

109. **c** Systems analysis is generally the first step in the systems development life cycle after the decision to implement the system has been made. It helps determine the needs for data, storage, reporting, and functionality (Sayles and Trawick 2014, 74).

110. **b** The mean is sensitive to extreme measures. That is, it is strongly influenced by outliers (Horton 2016, 221–222).

111. **c** The Federated—inconsistent databases—model for HIE includes multiple enterprises agreeing to connect and share specific information in a point-to-point manner (Amatayakul 2017, 417–418).

112. **d** A basic service provided by an HIE organization must be the actual transmission of the data. This is the technical networking service that provides appropriate bandwidth, latency, availability, ubiquity, and security (Amatayakul 2017, 420).

113. **b** The data shows that Dr. Jones' outcomes are all higher than the OB/GYN group. This data indicates that Dr. Jones should be monitored for continued poor performance compared to his peer group (Shaw and Carter 2015, 349).

114. **b** Terminal digit filing is a common method of paper record filing. Records are filed according to a three-part number made up of two-digit pairs. Option b is correct because the order is established with the third, or terminal, two-digit pairs (Reynolds and Sharp 2016, 128–129).

115. **d** Challenges are those inevitable elements that pose barriers to achieving success with a health information system. Without recognizing them as early in the planning process as possible, it becomes very difficult to overcome them. An environmental scan is a process to formally identify challenges that considers both internal and external factors (Amatayakul 2016, 394–395).

116. **d** The use case is based on the organization's redesigned processes and ask the vendor how its products would perform the inherent functions. The approach is useful for avoiding yes and no responses (Amatayakul 2017, 189).

117. **a** The master patient index (MPI) is a permanent database including every patient ever admitted to or treated by the facility. Even though patient health records may be destroyed after legal retention periods have been met, the information contained in the MPI must be kept permanently (Reynolds and Sharp 2016, 129).

118. **a** Questionnaires allow for a large number of users to provide input about the needs of the system (Sayles and Trawick 2014, 75).

119. **c** Master patient index (MPI) contains patient-identifiable data such as name, address, date of birth, dates of hospitalizations or encounters, name of attending physician, and health record number (Reynolds and Sharp 2016, 130).

120. **c** Formal and informal mechanisms should be used to evaluate each vendor and its products. For example, the project team may hold vendor presentations, check references, attend user group meetings, and make site visits to other facilities that use the product. The purpose of these activities is to gather as much relevant information as possible to make an informed decision (Amatayakul 2017, 202–204).

121. **a** Data repositories in healthcare organizations require tools designed to perform intricate data searches and retrievals using online or real-time transaction processing (OLTP) (Amatayakul 2017, 306–307).

122. **a** The bar code symbol was standardized for the healthcare industry making it easier to adopt barcoding technology. Barcoding applications have been adopted for labels, patient wristbands, specimen containers, business/employee/patient records, library reference materials, medication packages, dietary items, paper documents, and more (Rinehart-Thompson 2016, 351).

123. **d** The clinician or physician web portals were first seen as a way for clinicians to easily access (via a web browser) the healthcare provider organizations' multiple sources of structured and unstructured data from any network-connected device. Like clinical workstations, clinician or physician web portals evolved into an effective medium for providing access to multiple applications as well as the data (Sandefer 2016a, 355).

124. **c** HIPAA mandates that healthcare-covered entities and business partners implement a common standard (ASC X12N) for the transfer of information and accept the standard-based electronic transaction. This regulation does not apply to the transfer of data and information within a healthcare organization, but it does apply to the transfer of data and information external to and between healthcare organizations (Sayles and Trawick 2014, 175).

125. **c** Hospital Compare reports on 139 measures of hospital quality of care for heart attack, heart failure, pneumonia, and the prevention of surgical infections. The data available at Hospital Compare is reported by hospitals to meet the requirements of the Medicare Value Based Purchasing program (White 2016a, 188).

126. **d** Once all requirements are determined for functionality, vendor strategy, and other elements being sought from a vendor, an organization typically compiles all of this information into a request for proposal (RFP). This solicitation to vendors usually also includes basic information about the healthcare organization, such as how many users will be using the system, the timeline for implementation, and any special contractual issues that must be addressed (Amatayakul 2016, 403).

127. **b** Bar charts are used to display data from one or more variables. The bars may be drawn vertically or horizontally. Bar charts are used for nominal or ordinal variables. In this case, you would be displaying the average length of stay by service and then within each service have a bar for each hospital (Horton 2016, 257–258).

128. **d** Predictive modeling applies statistical techniques to determine the likelihood of certain events occurring together. Statistical methods are applied to historical data to learn the patterns in the data. These patterns are used to create models of what is most likely to occur (White 2016a, 7; White 2016b, 531).

129. **b** Contingency tables are a useful method for displaying the relationship between two categorical variables. Contingency tables are often referred to by the number of rows and columns (White 2016a, 64).

Domain 4

130. **d** The quality of coded clinical data depends on a number of factors, including accuracy. Accuracy is ensuring that the coded data is free from error and a correct representation of the patient's diagnosis and procedures (Sharp and Madlock-Brown 2016, 197).

131. **b** During order-entry a unique identifier for each service is entered. This unique identifier triggers a charge from the chargemaster to be posted on the patient's account. This process is known as hard coding (Casto and Forrestal 2015, 253).

132. **d** Medical identity theft occurs when a patient uses another person's name and insurance information to receive healthcare benefits. Most often this is done so a person can receive medical care with an insurance benefit and pay less or nothing for the care he or she receives (Rinehart-Thompson 2016, 71).

133. **c** Unbundling is the practice of using multiple codes that describe individual components of a procedure rather than using an appropriate single code that describes all steps of the procedure performed. Unbundling is a component of the NCCI and is what the coder in this example was doing. The use of audits or other evaluation techniques to monitor compliance and assist in the reduction of identified problem areas and corporate compliance is necessary to become aware of coding issues and stop them. The coder would need to be educated regarding unbundling and would be advised to stop the practice immediately (Kuehn 2017, 36).

134. **d** In conjunction with the corporate compliance officer, the health information manager should provide education and training related to the importance of complete and accurate coding, documentation, and billing on an annual basis. Technical education for all coders should be provided. Documentation education is also part of compliance education. A focused effort should be made to provide documentation education to the medical staff. Coding is based primarily on physician documentation, so nursing staff would not be included in the education process (Hunt 2016, 288).

135. **c** Aging of accounts is maintained in 30-day increments (0–30 days, 31–60 days, and so forth) (Casto and Forrestal 2015, 255).

136. **d** When the claim is submitted the reviewer should compare all the diagnoses and procedures printed on the bill with the coded information in the health record system. This process will help identify whether the communication software between the health record system and the billing system is functioning correctly. The HIM department should share the results of this comparison with patient financial services and the information technology department (Casto and Forrestal 2015, 254).

137. **a** A query is a routine communication and education tool used to advocate for complete and compliant documentation. The query is directed to the provider who originated the progress note or other report in question. This could include the attending physician, consulting physician, or the surgeon. In most cases, a query for abnormal test results would be directed to the attending physician (Hunt 2016, 276–277).

138. **b** Nonparticipating providers (nonPARs) do not sign a participation agreement with Medicare but may or may not accept assignment. If the nonPAR physician elects to accept assignment, he or she is paid 95 percent (5 percent less than participating physicians). For example, if the MFS amount is $200, the PAR provider receives $160 (80 percent of $200), but the nonPAR provider receives only $152 (95 percent of $160). In this case, the physician is participating so he or she will receive 80 percent of the MFS or $240 (80 percent of $300) (Casto and Forrestal 2015, 153–154).

139. **a** The Medicare Audit Contractor (MAC) reviews prepayment and postpayment, automated, and complex types of reviews to prevent future improper payment. The Medicare Recovery Audit Contractors (RACs) review post-payment, automated, and complex reviews to detect and correct past improper payments. The Quality Improvement Organization (QIO) reviews inpatient hospital claims to prevent improper payment through DRG upcoding (Casto and Forrestal 2015, 38–39).

140. **d** Revenue cycle management is the supervision of all administrative and clinical functions that contribute to the capture, management, and collection of patient service revenue (Casto and Forrestal 2015, 252).

141. **d** The Joint Commission has five accreditation decision categories. One of these categories is Contingent Accreditation. Contingent Accreditation is when the organization fails to resolve the requirements of an Accreditation with a follow-up survey. Although organizations that receive contingent accreditation may appeal, they must also remedy the noncompliance to the satisfaction of the Commission and, in most cases, are subject to a follow-up survey in 30 days (Shaw and Carter 2015, 418).

142. **a** The focused review indicated areas of risk related to lower weighted MS-DRGs from triple and pair combinations which may be the result of a coder missing secondary diagnoses. A focused audit based on this specific potential problem area could help to identify these cases. Optimization seeks the most accurate documentation, coded data, and resulting payment in the amount the provider is rightly and legally entitled to receive (Hunt 2016, 286).

143. **b** The Department of Veterans Affairs provides covered healthcare services and supplies to eligible beneficiaries through the Civilian Health and Medical Program of the Department of Veterans Affairs (CHAMPVA). This benefits program is available for the spouse or widow(er) and for the children of a veteran who meet certain criteria (Casto and Forrestal 2015, 92).

144. **d** It is not appropriate for the coder to assume that the removal was done by either snare, ablation, or hot biopsy forceps. The coding professional must query the physician to assign the appropriate code (Hunt 2016, 276–277).

145. **a** Accreditation is the act of granting approval to a healthcare organization. The approval is based on whether the organization has met a set of voluntary standards that were developed by the accreditation agency. The Joint Commission is an example of an accreditation agency (Shaw and Carter 2015, 406).

146. **c** Late charges are any charges that have not been posted to the account number within the healthcare facility's established bill hold time period. By incorporating this predicted billing delay into normal operations, the facility creates a preventive control to avoid under billing or having to submit late charges to the payer. For the provider to be paid for these charges, an adjusted claim must be sent to Medicare (Malmgren and Solberg 2016, 248).

147. **c** Once the claim is submitted to the third-party payer for reimbursement, the accounts receivable clock begins (Casto and Forrestal 2015, 255).

148. **c** Medicare or Medicaid certification programs are conducted by state licensure agencies working under contract with the Centers for Medicare and Medicaid Services (CMS). Hospitals must undergo Medicare and Medicaid certification surveys annually if they do not qualify for deemed status. Such facilities may have chosen to NOT participate in one of the accreditation programs that have deemed status recognition by CMS (James 2013c, 447).

149. **d** Hospitals have invested in clinical documentation improvement (CDI) programs to assure the health record accurately reflects the actual condition of the patient. Some of the goals of a CDI program include: identifying and clarifying missing, conflicting, or nonspecific physician documentation related to diagnosis and procedures; promoting health record completion during the patient's course of care; and improving communication between physicians and other members of the healthcare team (Hunt 2016, 268).

150. **a** In the outpatient setting, do not code a diagnosis documented as "probable." Rather, code the conditions to the highest degree of certainty for the encounter (Schraffenberger and Palkie 2017, 102).

151. **b** Focused selections of coded accounts are necessary for deeper understanding of patterns of error or change in high-risk areas or other areas of specific concern. Optimization seeks the most accurate documentation, coded data, and resulting payment in the amount the provider is rightly and legally entitled to receive (Hunt 2016, 286).

152. **c** During a clinical documentation improvement quality review, an organization should track and monitor the following elements: validity of queries generated, validity of working DRG assignment, validity of CDI specialist's assignment, and missed query opportunities (Hess 2015, 210).

153. **d** A claim lists the fees or charges for each service (Casto and Forrestal 2015, 9).

Domain 5

154. **a** Knowledge of the internal and external environment is essential to vision and strategy formulation. An environmental assessment is defined as a thorough review of the internal and external conditions in which an organization operates. This data-intensive process is the continuous process of gathering and analyzing intelligence about trends that are—or may be—affecting an organization and industry. IBM did not see the market demands and change in the personal home computing environment quickly enough, so their competitors were out to market ahead of them (McClernon 2016, 933).

155. **a** A permanent variance is a financial term that refers to the difference between the budgeted amount and the actual amount of a line item that is not expected to reverse itself during a subsequent period (Revoir and Davis 2016, 861–862).

156. **d** First calculate the number of productive hours in a day: 88% × 8 hours = 7.04 hours/day. Then determine the number of records filed per record filer: 1,000 / 3 = 333.3. Then divide 333 records / 7 hours = 47.5 or 48 charts/hour per productive FTE (Oachs 2016, 805–806).

157. **a** Every aspect of management involves a strategic management component. With organizational learning as a centerpiece, this approach unifies change management, strategy development, and leadership. In all three, people learn by observing and reflecting on the results of experiences (Revoir and Davis 2016, 930).

158. **c** Ground rules must be agreed upon by the team at the very beginning of the process improvement effort. All members of the team should have input into the ground rules. They should agree to abide by them for the sake of the team's success (Shaw and Carter 2015, 63–64).

159. **c** Strategic planning is a formalized roadmap that describes how the company executes the chosen strategy. A strategic plan spells out where an organization is going over the next three to five years and how it is going to get there. HIM professionals can use strategy to shape and influence change in their department and organization (McClernon 2016, 928).

160. **b** Employers acknowledge the need for mental health services for their employees by providing access to employee assistance programs (EAPs). These outpatient programs are designed to provide employees with immediate access to psychological counseling on a limited basis and may be provided on-site or through local providers (Munn 2013, 609).

161. **d** The discipline of ergonomics has helped redefine the employee workspace with consideration for comfort and safety (Oachs 2016, 790).

162. **a** The rectangle symbol in a flowchart is called a process icon and represents periods in the process when actions are being performed by human participants (Shaw and Carter 2015, 198).

163. **a** Sound change strategies and tactics alone do not ensure success. Success depends on great execution, including securing support for the needed organizational change efforts (Shaw and Carter 2015, 470).

164. **d** Conflict management focuses on working with the individuals involved to find a mutually acceptable solution. There are three ways to address conflict: compromise, control, and constructive confrontation. Constructive confrontation is a method in which both parties meet with an objective third party to explore their perceptions and feelings. The desired outcome is to produce a mutual understanding of the issues and to create a win-win situation (LeBlanc 2016, 744).

165. **a** The Hay Guide Chart-Profile Method of Job Evaluation is widely used as a job evaluation tool (LeBlanc 2016, 740).

166. **b** The elements of a contract must be stated clearly and specifically. A contract cannot exist unless all the following elements exist: there must be an agreement between two or more persons or entities and the agreement must include a valid offer, acceptance, and exchange of consideration (Rinehart-Thompson 2016, 56).

167. **d** Quantity standards (also called productivity standards) and quality standards (also known as service standards) are generally used by managers to monitor individual employee performance and the performance of a functional unit or the department as a whole. To properly communicate performance standards, managers need to make the distinction between quantitative and qualitative standards and identify examples of each for the HIS functions (Oachs 2016, 800).

168. **c** Delegation is the process of distributing work duties and decision making to others. To be effective, delegation should be commensurate with authority and responsibility. A manager must assign responsibility, which is an expectation that another person will perform tasks. At the same time, authority, or the right to act in ways necessary to carry out assigned tasks, must be granted (LeBlanc 2016, 738).

169. **d** If one thing can be accurately predicted about a project, it is that it will not progress as scheduled. To account for the inevitable changes, the project manager should be aware of the potential risks of the project and may need to adjust the project schedule, work effort, or cost projections to manage any anticipated risk (Olson 2016, 905–907).

170. **b** The net income is based only on the arithmetic difference between total revenue and total expenses of the current fiscal year. The difference between the total revenue of $2,500,000 and the total expenses of $2,250,000 is $250,000 (Revoir and Davis 2016, 849).

171. **d** In a not-for-profit environment, the difference between assets and liabilities is referred to as net assets. These relationships can be expressed in the following equation:

$$\text{Assets} - \text{Liabilities} = \text{Net assets (equity)}$$

In this example, add the assets (cash $500,000 + A/R $250,000 + building $1,000,000 + land $700,000 = $2,450,000) and then subtract the liabilities (A/P $350,000 + mortgage $600,000 = $950,000) or $2,450,000 – $950,000 = $1,500,000 (Revoir and Davis 2016, 842–843).

172. **d** The payback period is the time required to recoup the cost of an investment. Mortgage refinancing analysis frequently uses the concept of payback period. Mortgage refinancing is considered when interest rates have dropped. Refinancing may require up-front interest payments, called points, as well as a variety of administrative costs. In this example, the payback period is the time it takes for the savings in interest to equal the cost of the refinancing. For this problem, it is asking how long it will take to pay back the money spent to refinance. The hospital is spending $12,000 to refinance and will save $500 a month once they do. The payback period, or time to recoup their costs, is $12,000/ $500 = 24 months or two years (Revoir and Davis 2016, 866–867).

173. **a** The foundations of care giving, which include buildings (environmental services), equipment (technical services), professional staff (human resources), and appropriate policies (administrative systems) are examples of system performance measurements. Fifty percent of an HIM department's staff having a nationally recognized credential would be an example of a performance measure in the system (Shaw and Carter 2015, 44).

174. **b** Basic work distribution data can be collected in a work distribution chart, which is initially filled out by each employee and includes all responsible task content. Task content should come directly from the employee's current job description. In addition to task content, each employee tracks each task's start time, end time, and volume or productivity within a typical workweek. The results of a work distribution analysis can lead a department to redefine the job descriptions of some employees, redesign the office layout, or establish new or revised procedures for some department functions in order to gain improvements in staff productivity or service quality (Oachs 2016, 792).

175. **d** One of the most significant changes during a project is a change to the project scope. Various stakeholders frequently wish to add new or enhanced project requirements after the initial requirements were gathered, and the schedule and budget were established based on these requirements. Over time, these small changes in scope create significant changes and require more resources and time than originally planned. These incremental changes are commonly referred to as scope creep (Olson 2016, 905).

176. **c** Videoconferencing permits additional flexibility in delivering courses that may be enhanced through visual as well as audio presentation, such as those that include demonstrations or simulation exercises. Videoconferencing is useful for training employees in organizations with multiple sites, such as integrated delivery networks with inpatient and outpatient facilities. The expense is justified for large organizations that do extensive training (Patena 2016, 775).

177. **c** Releasing accurate information for public health purposes for patients with communicable diseases, such as AIDS or a venereal disease, and assisting with the complexities of information management in the context of bioterrorism and the threat or reality of global diseases, such as smallpox or Avian flu, are ethical responsibilities of the HIM professional (Gordon and Gordon 2016, 922–923).

178. **b** Advocates of emotional intelligence believe that awareness and use of feelings complements rational intelligence and experience, and it is the combination of these that is the key to success (Swenson 2016, 682).

179. **a** As much as individuals differ in their responses to change, it should not be surprising that various departments, units, and professions as well as other stakeholders also can vary in their responses. The level of perceived impact on organizational and unit culture as well as effect on work styles and turf can dramatically affect responses. For example, in some departments where there is little direct impact, staff may experience minor disruption of daily work and status quo. On the other hand, those who are more affected may show a decline in productivity, have lower morale, and express more complaints. To account for the inevitable changes, the project manager should be aware of the potential risks of the project and may need to make adjustments (Swenson and Olson 2016, 713, 905–906).

180. **b** An EHR steering committee or project sponsorship may go by different names. Virtually every organization that undertakes an EHR project forms a steering committee of some type to initiate the project and gain representation from all stakeholders in product selection and implementation (Amatayakul 2017, 222).

Practice Question Answers

Domain 1

1. **c** Patients who are admitted for an HIV-related illness should be assigned a minimum of two codes in the following order: code B20 to identify the HIV disease and additional codes to identify the related diagnosis, which in this case is disseminated candidiasis code B37.7 (Schraffenberger and Palkie 2017, 123).

2. **a** Data are raw facts generally stored as characters, words, symbols, measurements, or statistics (Johns 2016, 78; AHIMA 2014, 42).

3. **d** Derived data consist of factual details aggregated or summarized from a group of health records that provide no means to identify specific patients. These data should have the same level of confidentiality as the legal health record. However, derived data should not be considered part of the legal health record and would not be produced in response to a court order, subpoena, or request for the health record (Fahrenholz 2013a, 39).

4. **d** Clinicians use health record information to develop clinical pathways and other clinical practice guidelines, which help clinicians make knowledge- and experience-based decisions on medical treatment. These guidelines make it easier to coordinate multidisciplinary care and services (Fahrenholz 2013b, 78).

5. **d** Appropriate documentation of health record destruction must be maintained permanently no matter how the process is carried out. This documentation usually takes the form of a certificate of destruction (Fahrenholz 2013b, 112).

6. **c** The root operation performed was resection—cutting out or off, without replacement, all of a body part. Even though the entire liver was not removed, the correct root operation is resection based on coding guideline B3.8. PCS contains specific body parts for anatomical subdivisions of a body part, such as lobes of the lungs and liver and regions of the intestine. Resection of the specific body part is coded whenever all of the body part is cut out or off, rather than coding Excision of a less specific body part. The correct code is 0FT20ZZ. The section is Medical and Surgical—character 0; Body System is Hepatobiliary and Pancreas—character F; Root Operation is Resection—character T; Body Part is Liver, Left Lobe—character 2; Approach is Open—character 0; No Device—character Z; and No Qualifier—character Z (Kuehn and Jorwic 2017, 9, 21–23, 45).

7. **b** Sepsis is a serious medical condition caused by the body's immune response to an infection. Code A41.01 is for sepsis with methicillin-susceptible *Staphylococcus aureus*. Because abdominal pain is a symptom of diverticulitis, only the diverticulitis of the colon is coded (Schraffenberger and Palkie 2017, 27, 119).

8. **d** The ICD-10-CM index entry for Diabetes, type 1, with gangrene provides E10.52 as the correct code, so the peripheral angiopathy is presumed when gangrene is present (Schraffenberger and Palkie 2017, 34).

9. **c** ICD-10-PCS coding guideline B3.4b states that if a diagnostic Excision, Extraction, or Drainage procedure (biopsy) is followed by a more definitive procedure, such as Destruction, Excision, or Resection at the same procedure site, both the biopsy and the more definitive treatment are coded (Kuehn and Jorwic 2017, 43).

10. **d** In physician practices, patients are informed of their option to transfer their records to another provider. The majority of complete contracts specify that health records are owned by the provider group (Rinehart-Thompson 2017c, 199–200).

11. **c** The data dictionary should be designed to accommodate changes resulting from clinical or technical advances and regulatory changes. There should be a plan for future expansion, such as expanding a data field from one element to multiple elements. This becomes problematic when comparing data across time if the meaning of a particular element has changed while its name or representation has not (Russo 2013b, 322).

12. **b** Examples of metadata include name of element, definition, application in which the data element is found, locator key, ownership, entity relationships, date first entered system, date terminated from system, and system of origin (Russo 2013b, 321–322).

13. **d** Biomedical research is considered an ancillary function of the health record (Fahrenholz 2013b, 85).

14. **a** Logical Observation Identifiers, Names and Codes (LOINC) is a well-accepted set of terminology standards that provide a standard set of universal names and codes for identifying individual laboratory and clinical results (Palkie 2016a, 155).

15. **d** The Uniform Ambulatory Care Data Set (UACDS) includes data elements specific to ambulatory care such as the reason for the encounter with the healthcare provider (Johns 2015, 280).

16. **b** Medicare requires that all inpatient hospitals collect a minimum set of patient-specific data elements, which are in databases formulated from hospital discharge abstract systems. The patient-specific data elements are referred to as the Uniform Hospital Discharge Data Set (UHDDS) (Russo 2013a, 295).

17. **b** Unstructured data is often preferred over structured data because it enables providers to document details and nuance that are usually not available with structured data (Biedermann and Dolezel 2017, 159).

18. **b** Care plans are required documentation in a long-term care hospital (LTCH). Some LTCHs may use critical paths (or clinical pathways) for specific patients (James 2013a, 520–521).

19. **b** Because of the risks associated with miscommunication, verbal orders are discouraged. When a verbal order is necessary, a clinician should sign, give his or her credential (for example, RN, PT, or LPN), and record the date and time the order was received. Verbal orders for medication are usually required to be given to, and to be accepted only by, nursing or pharmacy personnel (Rinehart-Thompson 2017c, 178).

20. **c** Auditing integrity: Inadequate auditing functions that make it impossible to detect when an entry was modified or borrowed from another source and misrepresented as an original entry by an authorized user (Russo 2013b, 338).

21. **d** The integrated health record is arranged so that the documentation from various sources is intermingled and follows a strict chronological or reverse-chronological order. The advantage of the integrated format is that it is easy for caregivers to follow the course of the patient's diagnosis and treatment (Russo 2013b, 305).

22. **b** The data flow for a hospital inpatient can begin in several ways. Data collection starts in the registration department if patients are a direct admission for their physician's office or hospital outpatient department. Data collection begins in the emergency room if the patients arrive at the hospital, are assessed in the emergency room, and are admitted as an inpatient. No matter where the data collection begins, the same patient demographic information is collected. During the course of the inpatient stay, patient care is delivered and data is captured. As care is delivered and procedures are performed, charges are entered either by nursing staff or the personnel performing the procedure. After the patient is discharged, diagnosis and procedure codes are assigned (White 2016a, 23–24).

23. **b** Quantitative analysis is a review of the health record to identify deficiencies to ensure completeness and accuracy. It is generally conducted retrospectively, that is, after the patient's discharge from the facility or at the conclusion of treatment (Reynolds and Sharp 2016, 123).

24. **b** Every long-term care facility must complete a comprehensive assessment of every resident's needs by using the resident assessment instrument (RAI) specified by the state in which the facility operates (James 2013b, 536–538).

25. **a** Data standards allow us to share data in a uniform way. Data standards include data content standards and data exchange standards. Data content standards are clear guidelines for the acceptable values for specified data fields. The use of data content standards make it possible to share information so that users are able to interpret data in the same way (Sayles and Trawick 2014, 55).

26. **c** Computer-assisted coding (CAC) cannot address the major obstacle facing today's human coder: the lack of accurate, complete clinical documentation (Hunt 2016, 281).

27. **a** There are many types of patient-identifiable data elements that are pulled from the patient's healthcare record that are not included in the legal health record or designated record set definitions. Administrative data and derived data and documents are two examples of patient-identifiable data that are used in the healthcare organization. Administrative data are patient-identifiable data used for administrative, regulatory, healthcare operation, and payment (financial) purposes (Fahrenholz 2013a, 62).

28. **b** For elective hospital admissions, the patient or the admitting physician's office staff often provide administrative information and demographic data before the patient comes to the hospital. Alternatively, the patient may provide the information to the hospital's registration staff on the day of admission or through a secure page of the organization's website prior to admission. In the case of an unplanned admission, the patient or the patient's representative provides administrative information. A patient's name, age, and address would be considered administrative data (Fahrenholz 2013b, 75).

29. **c** An electronic signature is a unique personal identifier that is entered by the author of EHR documentation via electronic means. Benefits of the electronic signature include legibility and automatic dating and time stamping of entries. The possibility of documentation error, however, is not eliminated with electronic signature (Russo 2013b, 337).

30. **b** The correct root operation is extirpation—taking or cutting out solid matter from a body part. The earlier lithotripsy would have been fragmentation but was not successful in removing the calculus (Kuehn and Jorwic 2017, 91).

31. **c** The International Classification of Diseases, Tenth Revision, Clinical Modification (ICD-10-CM) Coordination and Maintenance (C&M) Committee is chaired by a representative from the NCHS and a representative from CMS. The committee is responsible for maintaining the United States' clinical modification version of the ICD-10-CM/PCS code sets. The C&M Committee holds two open meetings each year that serve as a public forum for discussing (but not making decisions about) proposed revisions to ICD-10-CM/PCS (Schraffenberger and Palkie 2017, xxxiii).

32. **a** An encoder is used to increase the accuracy and efficiency of the coding process. Although encoders can cite official coding guidelines and provide code optimization guidance, they require user interaction. Encoders promote accuracy as well as consistency in the coding of diagnoses and procedures (Russo 2013c, 412).

33. **b** When entries are made in the health record regarding a patient who is particularly hostile or irritable, general documentation principles apply, such as charting objective facts and avoiding the use of personal opinions, particularly those that are critical of the patient. The degree to which these general principles apply is heightened because a disagreeable patient may cause a provider to use more expressive and inappropriate language. Further, a hostile patient may be more likely to file legal action in the future if the hostility is a personal attribute and not simply a manifestation of his or her medical condition (Rinehart-Thompson 2017c, 179).

34. **c** The provider is responsible for ensuring the quality of the documentation of the healthcare record (Rinehart-Thompson 2017c, 177).

35. **d** A one-to-one relationship exists when an instance of an entity (a row or record) is associated with one instance of another entity, and vice versa. There is only one bed per patient and one patient per bed. One-to-one relationships are rare in logical-level data models because they often indicate a separate entity is unnecessary (Sayles and Trawick 2014, 56).

36. **b** Healthcare organizations need to be very clear about which abbreviations are not acceptable to use when writing or communicating medication orders. The organization's policy should also define whether or when the diagnosis, condition, or indication for use is included on a medication order (Shaw and Carter 2015, 248–249).

37. **c** According to the UHDDS definition, ethnicity should be recorded on a patient record as non-Spanish/Hispanic or Spanish/non-Hispanic, or unknown. The UHDDS has been revised several times since 1986 (Russo 2013a, 296).

38. **a** The repair of the hernia is not coded because it was not performed; however, code 0WJG0ZZ is assigned to describe the extent of the procedure, inspection of the peritoneal cavity based on ICD-10-PCS Guideline B3.3. The Z53.09 is also used to indicate the canceled procedure due to the contraindication. The code R00.1 is also added for the bradycardia that the patient developed during the procedure (Kuehn and Jorwic 2017, 42; Schraffenberger and Palkie 2017, 681).

39. **b** The content of the resident assessment instruments (RAIs) is used to collect the necessary information from and about the facility resident. The RAI consists of three basic components: The Minimum Data Set (MDS), the Care Area Assessment (CAA) process, and the RAI utilization guidelines (James 2013b, 536–538).

40. **c** Each individual who has been authorized to document in the EHR uses a unique personal identifier in the form of a code or password. Some systems may use a combination of a unique logon ID and password as a means to validate the author of the documentation (Russo 2013b, 337–338).

41. **d** Because of cost and space limitations, permanently storing paper-based health record documents is not an option for most hospitals. The destruction of patient-identifiable clinical documentation should be carried out in accordance with relevant federal and state regulations and organizational policy. Paper documents can be destroyed by pulverizing, pulping, burning, or shredding as these are acceptable forms of destruction for that medium. Degaussing is an acceptable form of destruction of electronic documents (Fahrenholz 2013b, 111).

42. **b** Begin with the main term: Biopsy, artery, temporal (Kuehn 2017, 17–18, 22, 24).

43. **d** If the diagnosis documented at the time of discharge is qualified as "probable," "suspected," "likely," "questionable," "possible," or "still to be ruled out," or other similar terms indicating uncertainty, code the condition as if it existed or was established (Schraffenberger and Palkie 2017, 95).

44. **d** Modifier –24 is used for unrelated evaluation and management service by the same physician, or other qualified healthcare professional, during a postoperative period (Kuehn 2017, 50).

45. **c** The concept of legal health records (LHRs) was created to describe the data, documents, reports, and information that comprise the formal business records of any healthcare organization that are to be utilized during legal proceedings (Biedermann and Dolezel 2017, 424).

46. **c** In the hospital setting, data should conform to one of two uniform healthcare data sets: the uniform hospital discharge data set (UHDDS) for inpatient services and the uniform ambulatory care data set (UACDS) for outpatient services (Russo 2013a, 187).

47. **a** Present on admission is defined as present at the time the order for inpatient admission occurs—conditions that develop during an outpatient encounter, including emergency department, observation, or outpatient surgery, are considered present on admission. This patient was not admitted with a catheter-associated urinary infection, so that condition cannot be coded as present on admission (POA). The patient was admitted with symptoms of a stroke and diagnoses of COPD and hypertension. The CVA was documented after admission, but the symptoms of the stroke were POA, so this condition would be coded as POA (Schraffenberger and Palkie 2017, 85).

48. **d** Ongoing record review is a continuous health record quality review process. Clinical or HIM professionals review the records of current inpatients or outpatients to ensure that health records are complete and accurate and that the facility's clinical documentation practices meet relevant accreditation standards, state licensing laws, and federal regulatory requirements. Ongoing record reviews also address quality and patient safety initiatives by improving documentation practices (Russo 2013c, 425).

49. **b** The purpose of the data dictionary is to standardize definitions and ensure consistency of use. Standardizing data enhances use across systems. Communication is improved in clinical treatment, research, and business processes through a common understanding of terms (Russo 2013c, 321).

50. **c** An entity relationship diagram (ERD) is used to describe how the tables work together. The diagram is a graphic representation of the entities, attributes, and relationships that are part of a database and is a data modeling tool (White 2016a, 46).

51. **b** When erroneous entries are made in health records, written procedures should have provisions for how corrections are made. Educating clinicians who are authorized to document in the health record on the appropriate way to make corrections will promote consistency and standardization and maintain the integrity of the health record. Errors corrected in the paper-based record may be easier to identify visually than those corrected in electronic documentation systems (Russo 2013c, 343).

52. **a** Auto-authentication methods, which allow users to sign multiple documents at one time without opening the documents, do not require author review and therefore fall short of federal and state authentication requirements and place the organization at legal risk. Some providers choose not to enter their own progress notes electronically and instead use scribes or assistants to type entries into the system for subsequent authorization. Policies, procedures, and checks and balances must be in place to ensure that the physician or legally responsible individual reviews the health record entries and affixes an authorization compliant with existing law (Russo 2013c, 339).

53. **a** Code 54401 is correct because the prosthesis is self-contained (Kuehn 2017, 17–18, 22, 24).

54. **a** A simple query statement using the data manipulation language has three parts. The "select" statement is always first. This determines the label, or field name, of the data that is being retrieved (White 2016a, 48).

55. **b** Providers must have a process in place for handling amendments, corrections, and deletions in health record documentation. An amendment is an alteration of the health information by modification, correction, addition, or deletion (Biedermann and Dolezel 2017, 448).

56. **b** A database is a tool used to collect, retrieve, report, and analyze data. A database cannot function without a database management system (DBMS) to manipulate and control the data stored within the database. Databases allow data to be stored in one place and accessed by many different systems. This reduces the redundancy of data and improves data consistency. The decrease in redundancy leads to improved data quality, which in turn saves time by reducing the duplication of data entry (Sayles and Trawick 2014, 49–50).

57. **d** Authentication is the process of identifying the source of health record entries by attaching a handwritten signature, the author's initials, or an electronic signature and also the proof of authorship that ensures, as much as possible, that log-ins and messages from a user originate from an authorized source (Fahrenholz and Russo 2013, 688).

58. **a** Disaster recovery planning is the technological aspect of business continuity planning. HIM professionals assist in designing disaster recovery plans that address documenting information in the health record during down time or a disaster (Russo 2013b, 346–347).

59. **b** A monthly summary may be completed in the long-term care setting to help summarize the care given to the resident over time. There are no federal requirements for a summary note; however, state laws may be more specific. The monthly summary is a mechanism to capture concise monthly updates reflecting gains and declines in the resident's condition and health status. The monthly summary should correlate with the resident's care planning process and further support the MDS assessments (James 2013b, 543).

60. **b** Regardless of the healthcare setting, healthcare organizations must meet regulatory and accreditation standards when collecting and storing health information. These standards require a separate health record for each individual patient and address minimum documentation requirements to ensure that these records provide for continuity of patient care among providers (Fahrenholz 2013a, 25).

61. **c** A migration path is a strategic plan but is somewhat different than the traditional IT strategic plan that focuses only on applications and technology. The migration path should identify specific, measurable goals along a realistic timeline given the organization's current culture, information technology infrastructure, financial capability, and other strategic imperatives (Amatayakul 2016, 395).

62. **b** The hospital must have a medical record service that has administrative responsibility for medical records. A health record must be maintained for every individual evaluated or treated in the hospital. Health records must be retained in their original or legally reproduced form for a period of at least 5 years (James 2013a, 444).

63. **d** An advance directive (also called healthcare directive, advance healthcare directive, living will, or healthcare directive) is a legal document used to specify whether the patient would like to be kept on artificial life support if she becomes permanently unconscious or is otherwise dying and unable to speak for herself (James 2013b, 535).

64. **d** The destruction of patient-identifiable clinical documentation should be carried out in accordance with relevant federal and state regulations and organizational policy. Electronic data can be destroyed with magnetic degaussing (demagnetizing) as this is an acceptable form of destruction for that medium. Burning, shredding, and pulverizing are acceptable destruction methods for paper-based records (Fahrenholz 2013b, 111–112).

65. **b** Delinquent health records are those records that are not completed within the specified time frame, for example, within 14 days of discharge. A delinquent record is similar to an overdue library book. The definition of a delinquent chart varies according to the facility, but most facilities require that records be completed within 30 days of discharge as mandated by CMS regulations and Joint Commission standards. Some facilities require a shorter time frame for completing records because of concerns about timely billing (Reynolds and Sharp 2016, 126).

66. **a** Birth defects registries collect information on newborns with birth defects. Often population based, these registries serve a variety of purposes. For example, they provide information on the incidence of birth defects to study causes and prevention of birth defects, to monitor trends in birth defects to improve medical care for children with birth defects, and to target interventions for preventable birth defects such as folic acid to prevent neural tube defects (Sharp and Madlock-Brown 2016, 177).

67. **c** Templates often provide clinical information by default and design. When used inappropriately, they may misrepresent a patient's condition and might not reflect changes in a condition. Unless the physician or other authorized provider removes the default documentation from the visit note, a higher level of service than is actually provided could be assigned. All templates and autogenerated entries, such as laboratory results, have the potential to be problematic. Accordingly, management oversight is necessary. Appropriate care must be taken that the data captured and stored are accurate, complete, and associated with the correct patient record and encounter (Russo 2013b, 341).

68. **b** Data definition stewards function in a business, as opposed to a technical role; major responsibilities include identifying the specific data needed to operate business processes, recording business definitions and metadata, identifying and enforcing quality standards, communicating data issue concerns, and communicating new or changed business requirements (Johns 2016, 93).

69. **c** Data management is based on the assumption that all data have a life cycle. Typical data life cycle functions requiring data governance include: establishing what data are to be collected and how they are to be captured; setting standards for data retention and storage; determining processes for data access and distribution; establishing standards for data archival and destruction (Johns 2016, 82).

70. **c** Hybrid health records are increasingly seen as the most common transition points between fully paper and completely electronic records. Hybrid records may be a mixture of paper and electronic or multiple electronic systems that do not communicate or are not logically architected for record management (Biedermann and Dolezel 2017, 429).

71. **b** The HIM professional should be aware of the specific requirements for submitting discharge data using the uniform data set in the state where he or she practices. For those states that require mandatory reporting, the data sets collected by different hospitals can be compared, and the data can be combined for national analysis and healthcare delivery planning (Russo 2013a, 295).

72. **c** Immunization registries usually have the purpose of increasing the number of infants and children who receive proper immunizations at the proper intervals. To accomplish this goal, they collect information within a particular geographic area about children and their immunization status (Sharp and Madlock-Brown 2016, 180).

73. **d** Begin with the main term Revision; pacemaker site; chest (Kuehn 2017, 17–18, 22, 24).

74. **d** In a trauma registry, the case definition might be all patients admitted with a diagnosis falling into ICD-10-CM code numbers S00–T88, the trauma diagnosis codes (Sharp and Madlock-Brown 2016, 175–176).

75. **b** The one-to-many relationship exists when one instance of an entity is associated with many instances of another entity. If a physician may be linked to many patients and patients may only be related to one physician, this is an example of a one-to-many relationship (Sayles and Trawick 2014, 56).

76. **c** The health record is considered a primary data source because it contains patient-specific data and information about a patient that has been documented by the professionals who provided care or services to that patient (Fahrenholz 2013c, 159).

77. **c** Information governance is defined as ensuring leadership and organizational practices, resources, and controls for effective, compliant, and ethical stewardship of information assets to enable best clinical and business practices and serve patients, stakeholders, and the public good (Johns 2016, 79).

78. **a** In 1974, the federal government adopted the Uniform Hospital Discharge Data Set (UHDDS) as the standard for collecting data for the Medicare and Medicaid programs. When the Prospective Payment Act was enacted in 1983, UHDDS definitions were incorporated into the rules and regulations for implementing diagnosis-related groups (DRGs). A key component was the incorporation of the definitions of principal diagnosis, principal procedure, and other significant procedures, into the DRG algorithms (Russo 2013a, 295).

79. **d** Source-oriented is a system of health record organization in which information is arranged according to the patient care department that provided the care (Reynolds and Sharp 2016, 120).

80. **a** Secondary data sources provide information that is not readily available from individual health records. Data taken from health records and entered into disease-oriented databases can help researchers determine the effectiveness of alternative treatment methods and monitor outcomes (Fahrenholz 2013c, 159).

81. **a** Secondary data sources provide information that is not readily available from individual health records. Data taken from health records and entered into disease-oriented databases can help researchers determine the effectiveness of alternative treatment methods and monitor outcomes (Fahrenholz 2013c, 159).

82. **a** Common characteristics of data quality are relevancy, granularity, timeliness, currency, accuracy, precision, and consistency (Sharp and Madlock-Brown 2016, 197).

83. **d** Appropriate documentation of health record destruction must be maintained permanently no matter how the process is carried out. This documentation usually takes the form of a certificate of destruction (Fahrenholz 2013b, 112).

84. **a** Federal and state statutes, licensing requirements, and accreditation standards provide minimum guidelines to ensure accurate and complete documentation. Such documentation facilitates effective communication among caregivers to provide continuity of patient care, which is its primary purpose (Fahrenholz 2013a, 26).

85. **d** Quality has several components, including the following: appropriateness, the right care is provided at the right time; technical excellence, the right care is provided in the right manner; accessibility, the right care can be obtained when it is needed; and acceptability, the patients are satisfied (Fuller 2016, 28–29).

86. **d** The integrity of each piece of data, including any document, must be ensured to maintain highly defensible business records. Document and data nonrepudiation are the methods by which the data are maintained in an accurate form after their creation, free of unauthorized changes, modifications, updates, or similar changes (Biedermann and Dolezel 2017, 443).

87. **a** The physician index categorizes patients by primary physician. It guides the retrieval of cases treated by a particular physician. This index is created simply by sorting patients by physician (Fahrenholz 2013c, 156).

88. **b** Case finding includes the methods used to identify the patients who have been seen and treated in the facility for the particular disease or condition of interest to the registry. After cases have been identified, extensive information is abstracted from the health record and entered into the registry database (Sharp and Madlock-Brown 2016, 173).

89. **a** An object-oriented database is derived from object-oriented programming and has no single inherent structure. The structure for any given class or type of object can be anything a programmer finds useful—a linked list, a set, an array, etc. An object may contain different degrees of complexity, making use of multiple types and multiple structures (Amatayakul 2017, 306).

90. **b** Aggregate statistical data are also useful for clinical and administrative decision support. Indexes are used to sort data to assist with the study of certain data elements. HIM departments also collect and calculate various statistics about the operations of the healthcare facilities and clinical practices they serve (Fahrenholz 2013c, 152).

91. **d** A data dictionary is a descriptive list of the data elements to be collected in an information system or database whose purpose is to ensure consistency of terminology (Sharp and Madlock-Brown 2016, 196).

92. **d** Each facility must have a policy in place for dealing with situations where records remain incomplete for an extended period. The HIM director can be given authority to declare that a record is completed for purposes of filing when a provider relocates, dies, or has an extended illness that would prevent the record from ever being completed. Every effort should be made to have a partner or physician in the same specialty area complete the charts so that coding, billing, and statistical information are available (Reynolds and Sharp 2016, 104).

93. **a** The stakeholder team will drive the creation of the legal health record (LHR) documentation, undertake the LHR definition project, and be responsible for its continued maintenance. Establishment of the stakeholder team should be the first step in the LHR definition process (Biedermann and Dolezel 2017, 430).

94. **c** The Minimum Data Set for Long-Term Care is a federally mandated standard assessment form used to collect demographic and clinical data on nursing home residents. It consists of a core set of screening and assessment elements based on common definitions. To meet federal requirements, long-term care facilities must complete an MDS for every resident at the time of admission and at designated reassessment points throughout the resident's stay (James 2013b, 536).

95. **b** The National Committee on Vital and Health Statistics (NCVHS) has developed the initial efforts toward creating standardized data sets for use in different types of healthcare settings, including acute care, ambulatory care, long-term care, and home care (Fahrenholz 2013c, 155).

96. **a** Qualitative analysis is a review of the health record to ensure the adequacy of entries documenting the quality of care are present (Russo 2013c, 425).

97. **a** The continuity of care record (CCR) helps standardize clinical content for sharing between providers. A CCR allows documentation of care delivery from one healthcare experience to another (Sandefer 2016b, 436).

98. **b** In the case of a stillborn infant, often a separate patient record is not created—information is recorded in the mother's delivery record (Russo 2013a, 265).

99. **a** The sarcoma is an aberrant part of the soft tissue, which was removed. Although the physician documents this procedure as a resection, only part of the body part is removed. Coding guideline A11 states that it is the coder's responsibility to determine what the documentation in the medical record equates to in PCS definitions. This procedure would code to Excision. Excision is defined in ICD-10-PCS as cutting out or off, without replacement, a portion of a body part (Kuehn and Jorwic 2017, 39, 77).

100. **a** Regular reviews and updates of related policies and procedures to ensure the organization is always in compliance with the latest rules and trends in the legal health records (LHRs) is part of the LHR maintenance plan (Biedermann and Dolezel 2017, 432).

101. **c** Individual health records are a rich source of data about each patient. However, it is not easy to see trends in a population of patients by looking at individual records. To reveal patterns, data must be extracted from individual records and entered into databases (Fahrenholz 2013c, 152).

102. **d** The processes of storing health information and destroying it when it is no longer needed are called retention and destruction. The development of EHRs has given healthcare organizations the ability to retain and store health information without the physical space restriction of paper-based health records. These processes are subject to specific regulations in many states. Federal regulations and accreditation standards also include specific guidelines on the release and retention of patient-identified health information (Fahrenholz 2013a, 28).

103. **b** The newborn record would include the Apgar score, feeding and elimination status, weight, sleeping patterns, and head and chest measurements (Russo 2013a, 265–267).

104. **c** The technology used to support the EHR can provide many enhancements over the paper record. Technology also presents the potential for weakening the integrity of the information. One such risk occurs with the copy-and-paste forward functionality present in many operating systems and software programs (Biedermann and Dolezel 2017, 449).

105. **c** State laws, CMS regulations and other federal regulations, accreditation standards, and facility policies and procedures must also be reviewed when establishing a retention schedule. The HIM professional must adhere to the strictest time limit if the recommended retention period varies among different laws and regulations (Reynolds and Sharp 2016, 133).

Domain 2

106. **b** A license is required in order for medical students to practice medicine. Medical students must pass a test before they can obtain a license (Fuller 2016, 6).

107. **a** If physicians were to dictate information on patients they are treating in the facility, the disclosure of protected health information to the transcriptionists would be considered healthcare operations and, therefore, permitted under the HIPAA Privacy Rule. If physicians, who are separate covered entities, are dictating information on their private patients, however, it would be necessary for physicians to obtain a business associate agreement with the facility. It is permitted by the Privacy Rule for one covered entity to be a business associate of another covered entity (Thomason 2013, 26).

108. **b** Security audits are the mechanisms that record and examine activity in information systems. HIPAA does not specify what form of security audits must be used, how or how often they must be examined, or how long they must be retained (Brinda and Watters 2016, 322).

109. **c** The HIPAA Privacy Rule states that the covered entity must provide individuals with their information in the form that is requested by the individuals, if it is readily producible in the requested format. The covered entity can certainly decide, along with the individual, the easiest and least expensive way to provide the copies they request. Per the request of an individual, a covered entity must provide an electronic copy of any and all health information that the covered entity maintains electronically in a designated record set. If a covered entity does not maintain the entire designated record set electronically, there is not a requirement that the covered entity scan paper documents so the documents can be delivered electronically (Thomason 2013, 102).

110. **b** Original health records may be required by subpoena to be produced in person and the custodian of records is required to authenticate those records through testimony (Rinehart-Thompson 2017a, 59).

111. **a** The Professional Code of Ethics is based on ethical principles regarding privacy and confidentiality of patient information that have been an inherent part of the practice of medicine since the 4th century BC, when the Hippocratic Oath was created. Courts in various jurisdictions have concluded that a physician has a fiduciary duty to the patient to not disclose the patient's health and medical information (Theodos 2017, 14, 23).

112. **c** Patients (along with their next of kin or legal representatives) have the right to access their health records. However, health information management (HIM) professionals must validate the appropriateness of access. When a patient's next of kin or legal representative requests information belonging to the patient, HIM professionals should be familiar with state and federal laws regarding the right to access and who can authorize the use or disclosure of the information at issue (Fahrenholz 2013a, 29).

113. **c** The HIPAA Privacy Rule requires the covered entity to have business associate agreements in place with each business associate. This agreement must always include provisions regarding destruction or return of protected health information (PHI) upon termination of a business associate's services. Upon notice of the termination, the covered entity needs to contact the business associate and determine if the entity still retains any protected health information from, or created for, the covered entity. The PHI must be destroyed, returned to the covered entity, or transferred to another business associate. Once the PHI is transferred or destroyed, it is recommended that the covered entity obtain a certification from the business associate that either it has no protected health information, or all protected health information it had has been destroyed or returned to the covered entity (Thomason 2013, 18).

114. **d** Credentialing is the process that requires the verification of the educational qualifications, licensure status, and other experience of healthcare professionals who have applied for the privilege of practicing within a healthcare facility (Fahrenholz 2013b, 89).

115. **a** Data integrity means that data should be complete, accurate, consistent and up-to-date. With respect to data security, organizations must put protections in place so that no one may alter or dispose of data in a manner inconsistent with acceptable business and legal rules (Johns 2015, 211)

116. **d** The Stark Law or Federal Physician Self-Referral Statute prohibits physicians from referring Medicare or Medicaid patients for certain designated health services to an entity in which the physician or a member of his immediate family has an ownership or investment interest, or with which he or she has a compensation arrangement, unless an exception applies (Bowman 2017, 447).

117. **c** The HIPAA Privacy Rule permits healthcare providers to access protected health information for treatment purposes. However, there is also a requirement that the covered entity provide reasonable safeguards to protect the information. These requirements are not easy to meet when the access is from an unsecured location, although policies, medical staff bylaws, confidentiality or other agreements, and a careful use of new technology can mitigate some risks (Thomason 2013, 46).

118. **b** The HIPAA Privacy Rule allows communications to occur for treatment purposes. The preamble repeatedly states the intent of the rule is not to interfere with customary and necessary communications in the healthcare of the individual. Calling out a patient's name in a waiting room, or even on the facility's paging system, is considered an incidental disclosure and, therefore, allowed in the Privacy Rule (Thomason 2013, 37).

119. **c** Firewalls are hardware and software security devices situated between the routers of a private and public network. They are designed to protect computer networks from unauthorized outsiders (Sandefer 2016a, 366).

120. **c** Timely response is an important part of the Privacy Rule. A covered entity must act on an individual's request for review of PHI no later than 30 days after the request is made, extending the response by no more than 30 days if within the 30 day time period it gives the reasons for the delay and the date by which it would respond (Rinehart-Thompson 2017, 245).

121. **a** It is generally agreed that Social Security numbers (SSNs) should not be used as patient identifiers. The Social Security Administration is adamant in its opposition to using the SSN for purposes other than those identified by law. AHIMA is in agreement on this issue due to privacy, confidentiality, and security issues related to the use of the SSN (Fahrenholz 2013b, 76).

122. **a** The Privacy Rule states that an individual has a right of access to inspect and obtain a copy of his or her own PHI that is contained in a designated record set, such as a health record. The individual's right extends for as long as the PHI is maintained (Rinehart-Thompson 2017e, 243–244).

123. **b** Physical safeguards have to do with protecting the environment, including ensuring applicable doors have locks that are changed when needed and that fire, flood, and other natural disaster preparedness is in place (for example, fire alarms, sprinklers, smoke detectors, raised cabinets). Other physical controls include badging and escorting visitors and other typical security functions such as patrolling the premises, logging equipment in and out, and camera-monitoring key areas. HIPAA does not provide many specifics on physical facility controls but does require a facility security plan with the expectation that these matters will be addressed (Biedermann and Dolezel 2017, 390).

124. **c** One of the most fundamental terms in the Privacy Rule is PHI, defined by the rule as "individually identifiable health information that is transmitted by electronic media, maintained in electronic media, or transmitted or maintained in any other form or medium" (45 CFR 160.103). To meet the individually identifiable element of PHI, information must meet all three portions of a three-part test. (1) It must either identify the person or provide a reasonable basis to believe the person could be identified from the information given. (2) It must relate to one's past, present, or future physical or mental health condition; the provision of healthcare; or payment for the provision of healthcare. (3) It must be held or transmitted by a covered entity or its business associate (Rinehart-Thompson 2017d, 213).

125. **c** The HIPAA Security Rule requires covered entities to ensure the confidentiality, integrity, and availability of ePHI. The Security Rule contains provisions that require covered entities to adopt administrative, physical, and technical safeguards (Reynolds and Brodnik 2017a, 266–267).

126. **c** An EHR can provide highly effective access controls to meet the HIPAA Privacy Rule minimum necessary standard requirements. Role-based access controls are used where only specific classes of persons (for example, nurses) may access protected health information (Amatayakul 2017, 376–377).

127. **d** Firewalls are hardware and software security devices situated between the routers of a private and public network. They are designed to protect computer networks from unauthorized outsiders. However, they also can be used to protect entities within a single network, for example, to block laboratory technicians from getting into payroll records. Without firewalls, IT departments would have to deploy multiple-enterprise security programs that would soon become difficult to manage and maintain (Sandefer 2016a, 366).

128. **b** State laws have developed requirements for certain deaths, such as accidental, homicidal, suicidal, sudden, and suspicious in nature to be reported, usually to the medical examiner or coroner. In addition, deaths as a result of abortion or induced termination of pregnancy are also reportable (Brodnik 2017c, 392–393).

129. **a** The implementation of the Health Insurance Portability and Accountability Act (HIPAA) Privacy Rule in 2003 established a consistent set of privacy and security rules. These rules, designed to protect the privacy of patients, also attempted to simplify the sharing of health information for legitimate purposes. For example, before implementation of HIPAA, a healthcare provider who needed access to a health record maintained by another provider usually could not directly request the information. The former provider required the patient's written authorization to release information to the current provider. In many cases, the patient or the patient's legal representative had to facilitate the transfer of medical information to a current healthcare provider. Under federal privacy regulations, the healthcare provider can directly request protected medical information, and a written authorization from the patient is not required when the information is used for treatment purposes. The privacy rule states that protected health information used for treatment, payment, or healthcare operations does not require patient authorization to allow providers access, use, or disclosure. However, only the minimum necessary information needed to satisfy the specified purpose can be used or disclosed. The release of information for purposes unrelated to treatment, payment, or healthcare operations still requires the patient's written authorization (Fahrenholz 2013a, 27).

130. **a** An EHR can provide highly effective access controls to meet the HIPAA Privacy Rule minimum necessary standard requirements. Role-based access controls are used where only specific classes of persons may access protected health information. Context-based access controls add the dimensions that control not only class of persons but specific categories of information and under specific conditions for which access is permitted (Amatayakul 2017, 376–377).

131. **c** The facility access control standard requires covered entities to control and validate a person's access to a facility including visitor control (Biedermann and Dolezel 2017, 390–391).

132. **b** Administrative safeguards are administrative actions such as policies and procedures and documentation retention to manage the selection, development, implementation, and maintenance of security measures to safeguard ePHI and manage the conduct of the covered entities or business associates' workforce (Biedermann and Dolezel 2017, 383).

133. **d** The notice of privacy practices must explain and give examples of the uses of the patient's health information for treatment, payment, and healthcare operations, as well as other disclosures for purposes established in the regulations. If a particular use of information is not covered in the notice of privacy practices, the patient must sign an authorization form specific to the additional disclosure before his or her information can be released. Patient signature and e-mail address are not part of the notice of privacy practices (Reynolds and Sharp 2016, 105–106).

134. **b** Confidentiality is a legal ethical concept that establishes the healthcare provider's responsibility for protecting health records and other personal and private information from unauthorized use or disclosure (Brodnik 2017a, 7–8).

135. **a** When an individual who is at or above the age of majority becomes incapacitated, either permanently or temporarily, another person should be designated to make decisions for that individual including decisions about the use and disclosure of the individual's PHI. Whoever serves as the incompetent adult's personal representative should, at minimum, hold the incompetent adult's durable power of attorney (DPOA) or durable power of attorney for healthcare decisions (DPOA-HCD) (Brodnik 2017b, 342).

136. **c** It is the responsibility of the treating provider, in this case the physician who will be performing the surgery, to obtain informed consent and it may not be delegated to some other person (Klaver 2017c, 141).

137. **b** The HIPAA Privacy Rule states that protected health information used for purposes of treatment, payment, or healthcare operations does not require patient authorization to allow providers access, use, or disclosure. However, only the minimum necessary information needed to satisfy the specified purpose can be used or disclosed (Rinehart-Thompson 2017d, 216–217).

138. **b** Audit trails are used to facilitate the determination of security violations and to identify areas for improvement. Their usefulness is enhanced when they include trigger flags for automatic, intensified review (Sandefer 2016a, 366).

139. **b** A subpoena is a direct command that requires an individual or a representative of an organization to appear in court or to present an object to the court (Fahrenholz 2013b, 94).

140. **b** HIPAA permits an individual to request that a covered entity make an amendment to PHI in a designated record set. However, the covered entity may deny the request if it determines that the PHI or the record was not created by the covered entity. In this scenario the history and physical was created by General Hospital. Mercy Hospital would be able to deny the request because they did not create the history and physical for this patient (Rinehart-Thompson 2013, 67).

141. **b** Protecting the security and privacy of data in the database is called authorization management. Two of the important aspects of authorization management are user access control and usage monitoring (Rob and Coronel 2009; Amatayakul 2017, 376–377).

142. **c** The Health Information Technology for Economic and Clinical Health Act (HITECH) shortened the time frame for an accounting of disclosures. Previously, an accounting had to include disclosures made during the previous six years. This has been shortened to disclosures made during the previous three years (Rinehart-Thompson 2013, 153).

143. **a** The mental health professional can disclose information without an authorization from the patient in the following situations:

- The patient brings up the issue of the mental or emotional condition
- The health professional performs an examination under a court order
- Involuntary commitment proceedings
- A legal "duty to warn" an intended victim when a patient threatens to harm an identifiable victim(s)
- The mental health professional believes that the patient is likely to actually harm the individual(s) (Brodnik 2017b, 347–348).

144. **c** Generally speaking, the age of majority is 18 years old or older. This is the legal recognition that an individual is considered responsible for, and has control over, his or her actions (Klaver 2017c, 152).

145. **b** The HIPAA Privacy Rule allows individuals to decide whether they want to be listed in a facility directory when they are admitted to a facility. If the patient decides to be listed in the facility directory, the patient should be informed that only callers who know his or her name will be given any of this limited information. Covered entities generally do not, however, have to provide screening of visitors or calls for patients because such an activity is too difficult to manage with the number of employees and volunteers involved in the process of forwarding calls and directing visitors. If the covered entity agreed to the screening and could not meet the agreement, it could be considered a violation of this standard of the Privacy Rule (Thomason 2013, 105).

146. **d** The Uniform Health Care Decisions Act suggests that decision-making priority for an individual's next-of-kin be as follows: spouse, adult child, parent, adult sibling, or if no one is available who is so related to the individual, authority may be granted to "an adult who exhibited special care and concern for the individual" (Klaver 2017c, 159–160).

147. **d** Many state laws allow a minor to be treated as an adult for drug or alcohol dependency and sexually transmitted diseases or be given contraceptives and prenatal care without parental or legal guardian consent. This gives minors the right to treatment and access of their health records as a competent adult (Brodnik 2017b, 343–344).

148. **a** Patients may sign in their names on a waiting room list, and if another patient sees it, that is considered an incidental disclosure. However, in determining the content of these sign-in lists, the healthcare provider must take reasonable precautions that the information is limited to the minimum necessary for the purpose (Thomason 2013, 38).

149. **c** Generally, a hospital is liable to patients for the torts of its employees (including nurses and employed physicians) under the doctrine of *respondeat superior* (Latin for "let the master answer"). Also referred to as vicarious liability, under this doctrine the hospital holds itself out as responsible for the actions of its employees, provided that these individuals were acting within the scope of their employment or at the hospital's direction at the time they conducted the tortious activity in question (Rinehart-Thompson 2017c, 106–107).

150. **a** Employees in departments such as the business office, information systems, HIM, and infection control, who are not involved directly in patient care, will vary in their need to access patient information. The HIPAA "minimum necessary" principle must be applied to determine what access employees should legitimately have to PHI (45 CFR 164.502 [b]; Brodnik 2017b, 345).

151. **b** Reporting requirements mandate notification to the individual whose information was breached, and in the case of breaches of more than 500 individuals' information, to the media and the Secretary of Health and Human Services (Biedermann and Dolezel 2017, 401).

152. **b** The physician would not have access to records of a patient he or she is not treating unless the physician is performing designated healthcare operations such as research, peer review, or quality management. Otherwise the physician would need to have an authorization from the patient (Brodnik 2017b, 345–346).

153. **a** Encryption and destruction are the technologies and methodologies for rendering protected health information unusable, unreadable, or indecipherable to authorized individuals in order to prevent a potential breach of PHI (Biedermann and Dolezel 2017, 401).

154. **b** Job shadowing should be limited to areas where the likelihood of exposure to PHI is very limited, such as in administrative areas. There is a provision in the Privacy Rule that permits students and trainees to practice and improve their skills in the healthcare environment; however, the context of this provision appears to imply that the students are already enrolled in a healthcare field of study and that they are under the supervision of the covered entity. Most covered entities require students to be trained on confidentiality and other requirements of the Privacy Rule, and job shadowing activities do not appear to apply in this exception (Thomason 2013, 41).

155. **d** Redisclosure of health information is of significant concern to the healthcare industry. As such, the HIM professional must be alerted to state and federal statutes addressing this issue. A consent obtained by a hospital pursuant to the Privacy Rule in 45 CFR 164.506(a)(5) does not permit another hospital, healthcare provider, or clearinghouse to use or disclose information. However, the authorization content required in the Privacy Rule in 45 CFR 164.508(c)(1) must include a statement that the information disclosed pursuant to the authorization may be disclosed by the recipient and thus is no longer protected (Rinehart-Thompson 2017d, 231–232).

156. **d** One of the specifications found within the consent for use and disclosure of information should state that the individual has the right to revoke the consent in writing, except to the extent that the covered entity has already taken action based on the consent. In this situation, the facility acted in good faith based on the prior authorization and therefore the release is covered under the Privacy Act (Rinehart-Thompson 2017d, 223).

157. **a** Outcomes of quality improvement studies may be used to evaluate a physician's application for continued medical staff membership and privileges to practice. These studies are usually conducted as part of the hospital's QI activities. These review activities are considered confidential and protected from disclosure (Shaw and Carter 2015, 489–490).

158. **c** Employers who may or may not be HIPAA-covered healthcare organizations may request patient information for a number of reasons, including family medical leave certification, return to work certification for work-related injuries, and information for company physicians. Patient authorization is required for such disclosures, except in some states the patient's employer, employer's insurer, and employer's and employee's attorneys do not need patient authorization to obtain health information for workers' compensation purposes (Brodnik 2017b, 345).

159. **a** News media personnel (and others) may have an interest in obtaining information about a public figure or celebrity who is being treated or about individuals involved in events that have cast them in the public eye. However, the media is not exempt from the restrictions imposed by the HIPAA facility directory requirement, and it is prudent for a healthcare organization to exercise even greater restraint than that mandated by the facility directory requirement with respect to the media. Parents of adult children and attorneys also need an authorization to receive patient records. A hospital may disclose health information to law enforcement when the suspected criminal conduct has resulted in a death (Brodnik 2017b, 365).

160. **c** The maintenance of policies and procedures implemented to comply with the Security Rule must be retained for six years from the date of its creation or the date when it was last in effect, whichever is later (Reynolds and Brodnik 2017a, 278–279).

161. **d** The implementation of the Health Insurance Portability and Accountability Act (HIPAA) Privacy Rule in 2003 established a consistent set of privacy and security rules. The Privacy Rule states that protected health information used for treatment, payment, or healthcare operations does not require patient authorization to allow providers access, use, or disclosure. However, only the minimum necessary information needed to satisfy the specified purpose can be used or disclosed. The release of information for purposes unrelated to treatment, payment, or healthcare operations still requires the patient's written authorization (Fahrenholz 2013a, 27).

162. **b** A notice of privacy practices must be available at the site where the individual is treated and must be posted in a prominent place where the patient can be reasonably expected to read it (Rinehart-Thompson 2017d, 219).

163. **b** The notice of privacy practices must explain and give examples of the uses of the patient's health information for treatment, payment, and healthcare operations, as well as other disclosures for purposes established in the regulations. If a particular use of information is not covered in the notice of privacy practices, the patient must sign an authorization form specific to the additional disclosure before his or her information can be released (Reynolds and Sharp 2016, 105–106).

164. **c** Per HIPAA, covered entities may require individuals to make their access requests in writing if it has informed them of this requirement. A covered entity must act on an individual's request within 30 days, and may extend the response just once by no more than 30 days as long as it responds within the initial 30-day window and gives the reason for the delay and a date by which it will respond (Rinehart-Thompson 2013, 61).

165. **c** There are certain circumstances where the minimum necessary requirement does not apply, such as to healthcare providers for treatment; to the individual or his or her personal representative; pursuant to the individual's authorization to the Secretary of the HHS for investigations, compliance review, or enforcement; as required by law; or to meet other Privacy Rule compliance requirements (Rinehart-Thompson 2017d, 234).

166. **c** The Confidentiality of Alcohol and Drug Abuse Patient Records Rule is a federal rule that applies to information created for patients treated in a federally assisted drug or alcohol abuse program and specifically protects the identity, diagnosis, prognosis, or treatment of these patients. The rule generally prohibits redisclosure of health information related to this treatment except as needed in a medical emergency or when authorized by an appropriate court order or the patient's authorization (Rinehart-Thompson 2016, 70).

167. **d** Because incident reports contain facts, hospitals strive to protect their confidentiality. To ensure incident report confidentiality, no copies should be made and the original must not be filed in the health record nor removed from the files in the department responsible for maintaining them, typically risk management or QI. Also no reference to the completion of an incident report should be made in the health record. Such a reference would likely render the incident report discoverable because it is mentioned in a document that is discoverable in legal proceedings (Rinehart-Thompson 2016, 72).

168. **c** No authorization is needed to use or disclose PHI for public health activities. Some health records contain information that is important to the public welfare. Such information must be reported to the state's public health service to ensure public safety (Brinda and Watters 2016, 315).

169. **b** A significant part of the administrative simplification process is the creation of standards for the electronic transmission of data (Rinehart-Thompson 2017d, 207).

170. **d** The key to defining PHI is that it requires the information to either identify an individual or provide a reasonable basis to believe the person could be identified from the information given. In this situation, the information relates to a patient's health condition and could identify the patient (Rinehart-Thompson 2017d, 214).

171. **c** The HIPAA Privacy Rule intent is to allow an individual to obtain copies of records for a fee that is reasonable enough that an individual could pay for it. The Privacy Rule requires that the copy fee for the individual be reasonable and cost based. It can only include the costs of labor for copying, and postage, when mailed. The commentary to the Privacy Rule expands upon this standard. If paper copies are made, the fee can include the cost of the paper. If electronic copies are made, the fee can include copies of the media used (Thomason 2013, 96; Brodnik 2017b, 372–373).

172. **b** The Security Rule defines technical safeguards as the technology and the policy and procedures for its use that protect ePHI and controls access to it. A covered entity must determine which security measures and technologies are reasonable and appropriate for implementation (Biedermann and Dolezel 2017, 393).

173. **c** The three methods of two-factor authentication are something you know, such as a password or PIN; something you have, such as an ATM card, token, or swipe/smart card; and something you are, such as a biometric fingerprint, voice scan, iris, or retinal scan (Sayles and Trawick 2014, 219).

174. **b** Pursuant to the Privacy Rule, the hospital may disclose health information to law enforcement officials without authorization for law enforcement purposes for certain situations, including situations involving a crime victim. Disclosure is made in response to law enforcement officials' request for such information about an individual who is, or is suspected to be, a victim of a crime (Brinda and Watters 2016, 315).

175. **a** Training in HIPAA policies and procedures regarding PHI is required for all workforce members to carry out their job functions appropriately. The training should be ongoing and documented for each employee (Biedermann and Dolezel 2017, 371)

176. **a** Legislation gives a patient the right to obtain an accounting of disclosures of PHI made by the covered entity in the six years or less prior to the request date. Mandatory public health reporting is not considered part of a covered entities' operations. As a result, these disclosures must be included in an accounting of disclosures (Rinehart-Thompson 2017e, 247–248).

177. **d** PHI may not be used or disclosed by a covered entity unless the individual who is the subject of the information authorizes the use or disclosure in writing or the Privacy Rule requires or permits such use or disclosure without the individual's authorization. In this situation, Dr. Lawson is a covered entity and thus releasing the names of his asthma patients to a pharmaceutical company requires the patients' authorization (Rinehart-Thompson 2017d, 225).

178. **d** Title II of HIPAA is the most relevant title to the management of health information, containing provisions relating to the prevention of healthcare fraud and abuse and medical liability reform, as well as administrative simplification. The Privacy Rule derives from the administrative simplification provision of Title II along with the HIPAA security regulations, transactions and code set standardization requirements, unique national provider identifiers, and the enforcement rule (Rinehart-Thompson 2017d, 207).

179. **b** If a fee is assessed for a request, the fee schedule must be consulted and an invoice prepared. The fee schedule should be regularly reviewed for compliance with the HIPAA Privacy Rule and applicable state laws. A system should be developed to determine situations in which fees are not assessed, when prepayment is required, and to implement collection procedures for delinquent payments following record disclosure (Brodnik 2017b, 372–373).

180. **a** HIPAA established consumers' right to access and amend their own health records (Fahrenholz 2013a, 28).

181. **d** Vendors who have a presence in a healthcare facility, agency, or organization will often have access to patient information in the course of their work. If the vendor meets the definition of a business associate (that is, it is using or disclosing an individual's PHI on behalf of the healthcare organization), a business associate agreement must be signed. If a vendor is not a business associate, employees of the vendor should sign confidentiality agreements because of their routine contact with and exposure to patient information. In this situation, Ready-Clean is not a business associate (Brodnik 2017b, 346).

182. **b** A covered entity is any provider of medical or other healthcare services or supplies who transmits any health information in electronic form in connection with a transaction for which HHS has adopted a standard (Rinehart-Thompson 2017d, 218).

183. **b** One of the four areas of concern in an EHR environment is patient identification and demographic accuracy. When automated demographic or registration entries generate erroneous patient identification, this can lead to patient safety and quality-of-care issues and enable fraudulent activity involving patient identity theft or providing unjustified care for profit (Russo 2013b, 339).

184. **a** Common practice for covered entities is to accept the request, but not to agree to the restrictions because of the legal implications to the covered entity should the restriction be violated. Instead, if there are valid reasons why the patient requests the restriction, covered entities implement steps in an attempt to restrict the information as best as their systems and processes allow. The covered entity responds to the patient by describing measures it has taken but does not guarantee that the information is protected against incidental or accidental disclosure (Thomason 2013, 106–107).

185. **c** Individuals whose protected health information (PHI) has been breached must be provided with the following information: a description of what occurred (including date of breach and date that breach was discovered); the types of unsecured PHI that were involved (such as name, SSN, DOB, home address, and account number); steps that the individual may take to protect himself or herself; what the entity is doing to investigate, mitigate, and prevent future occurrences; contact information for the individual to ask questions and receive updates (AHIMA 2009; Rinehart-Thompson 2017e, 250–251).

186. **c** An e-discovery plan should be prepared well in advance of litigation, and it should be tailored to the organization's needs as determined by its size, scope, and complexity (Russo 2013b, 346).

187. **d** Because minors are, as a general rule, legally incompetent and unable to make decisions regarding use and disclosure of their own healthcare information, this authority belongs to the minor's parent(s) or legal guardian(s) unless an exception applies. Generally, only one parent's signature is required to authorize the use or disclosure of a minor's PHI. In this case, the adoptive parents are the legal guardians of the minor (Brodnik 2017b, 343).

188. **c** The Privacy Rule's general requirement is that authorization must be obtained for uses and disclosures of PHI created for research that includes treatment of the individual. Public information, deidentified data, or data that is recorded by the investigation so that the subject cannot be directly identified or identified through links are not subject to the Common Rule (Rinehart-Thompson 2017e, 251–252).

189. **c** The final exception to reporting requirements for breaches of PHI is applicable when covered entities and business associates who made an inadvertent disclosure has reason to believe that the recipient of the PHI would not have been able to retain the information. In this example, the provider called the patient with a common name to discuss laboratory results and dialed the wrong phone number. Although the provider discussed the results with "John Smith," no hard copy results were sent to the wrong patient, it is reasonable to believe that the wrong John Smith could not "keep" the information (Biedermann and Dolezel 2017, 401).

190. **c** Most states require healthcare personnel to report suspected abuse of specified classes of individuals such as children, the elderly, and other vulnerable categories of individuals such as the mentally disabled (Rinehart-Thompson 2017c, 180).

191. **d** Access control mechanisms are an effective means of controlling what and how users gain access to an electronic health information system. To authenticate the legitimate user of ePHI, the user must be assigned a unique identifier. Because of the public nature of the log-on, there is a need to authenticate the identity of the user, commonly with a password. Password systems allow for easily remembered log-ons that are hard to crack (Amatayakul 2017, 376–377).

192. **d** The Business Record Exception is the rule under which a record is determined to not be hearsay if it was made at or near the time by, or from information transmitted by, a person with knowledge; it was kept in the course of a regularly conducted business activity; and it was the regular practice of that business activity to make the record (Klaver 2017a, 80).

193. **b** *Darling v. Charleston Community Memorial Hospital* (1965) is a landmark case that established a hospital's responsibility for patient care. Touching directly on quality are the issues of the facility's responsibility to have effective methods of credentialing in place and effective mechanisms for continuing medical evaluation. The facility is responsible for knowing whether the care it provides meets acceptable standards of care (Rinehart-Thompson 2017b, 106).

194. **d** A facility may maintain a facility directory of patients being treated. HIPAA's Privacy Rule permits the facility to maintain in its directory the following information about an individual if the individual has not objected: name, location in the facility, and condition described in general terms. This information may be disclosed to persons who ask for the individual by name. An authorization is not necessary for public health purposes, health oversight agencies, and other reporting that is required by law (Rinehart-Thompson 2017d, 226).

195. **d** Security audits can help a healthcare organization proactively ensure that the information it stores and maintains is only being accessed for the normal course of business (Brinda and Watters 2016, 322).

196. **d** Maintaining a procedure to track PHI disclosures has been a common practice in departments that manage health information. However, HIPAA provides for an accounting of disclosures that gives an individual the right to receive a list of certain disclosures that a covered entity has made. Some of the disclosures for which an accounting is not required include: to the individual to whom the information pertains, incidental to an otherwise permitted or required use or disclosure, and pursuant to an authorization. A disclosure would be required for patient information faxes to an erroneous fax number (Rinehart-Thompson 2013, 68).

197. **a** The Security Rule intentionally leaves the methods for conducting the required risk analysis to the discretion of the entity. Regardless of the methods selected for conducting and documenting risk analysis, the Security Rule does mandate several elements that must be included in the analysis. These are: define the scope of the risk analysis, data collection, identify and document potential threats and vulnerabilities, assess current security measures, determine the likelihood of threat occurrence, determine the potential impact of threat occurrence, determine the level of risk, finalize documentation, and perform review and updates to the risk assessment (Biedermann and Dolezel 2017, 383).

198. **c** Vulnerability is defined as an inherent weakness or absence of a safeguard that could be exploited by a threat. Vulnerabilities are grouped into either technical or nontechnical categories, with technical vulnerabilities reflecting inappropriate information systems protective methods (Biedermann and Dolezel 2017, 381).

199. **c** The device and media controls standard states that covered entities are to implement policies and procedures that govern the receipt and removal of hardware and electronic media that contain electronic protected health information, into and out of a facility, and the movement of these items within the facility. This implementation specification includes maintaining a record of the movements of the hardware and electronic media and presents a growing challenge in many healthcare organizations where mobile technology is increasing in use (Biedermann and Dolezel 2017, 392).

200. **c** As the healthcare industry moves toward EHRs and key evidence contained in other electronic documents such as e-mails, a new legal term has evolved: e-discovery. The US Supreme Court recently amended the Federal Rules of Civil Procedure to address the discovery of electronic records, creating a new paradigm with respect to the production of documents as a discovery method (Rinehart-Thompson 2017a, 54).

201. **d** A subpoena instructing the recipient to bring documents and other records with himself or herself to a deposition or to court is a subpoena *duces tecum* (Rinehart-Thompson 2017a, 59).

202. **a** Elements of a valid subpoena commonly include the name of the court from which the subpoena was issued; the caption of action (the names of the plaintiff and defendant); assigned case docket number; date, time, and place of requested appearance; the information commanded, such as testimony or the specific documents sought in a subpoena *duces tecum* and the form in which that information is to be produced; the name of the issuing attorney; the name of the recipient being directed to disclose the records; and the signature or stamp of the court. The subpoena does not need to be signed by both the plaintiff and the defendant (Rinehart-Thompson 2017a, 60).

203. **a** Individuals must be informed in the NPP that PHI may be used for this purpose. Fundraising materials must include instructions on how to opt out of receiving solicitations in the future. If the individual has opted out of fundraising, this is to be treated as a revocation and no further solicitations may be sent to that individual. Fundraising may target a department of service or treating physician. However, if a fundraising activity targets individuals based on diagnosis (for example, patients with kidney disease are targeted to raise funds for a new kidney dialysis center), prior authorization is required. HITECH has strengthened fundraising requirements (Rinehart-Thompson 2013, 71).

204. **c** Emergency patients must be made aware of their rights. Transfer and acceptance policies and procedures must be delineated to ensure facilities comply with the Emergency Medical Treatment and Active Labor Act (EMTALA) and state regulations regarding transfers (Reynolds and Sharp 2016, 117).

205. **b** Steps have been taken by the organization to secure laptops, tablets, and mobile devices, such as smartphones and flash drives, including memory wipe to erase all data, even in instance of media reuse (Biederman and Dolezel 2017, 393).

206. **a** Access controls are the technical policies and procedures used to control access to ePHI. Access controls must be used to provide users with rights and limitations on what they can do in a system containing ePHI. The specific technology is not mandated, but each user must have unique user identification (Sayles and Trawick 2014, 218).

207. **c** Text messaging is used in healthcare. Text messages tend to be more synchronous, and thus more immediate, than e-mailing because of their brevity and immediate display on device screens. The following are best practices for minimizing privacy and security breaches associated with text messaging: encrypt during transmission, avoid text messages to more than one patient that could compromise confidentiality, confirm the telephone number of the patient being communicated with to avoid errant text messages and to avoid responding to text messages that may have been sent by someone else (under the guise of the patient's identity), use telephone numbers that have been stored in memory. To routinely verify their continued validity, train staff on text messaging policies and procedures (Rinehart-Thompson 2013, 134–135).

208. **a** Every member of the covered entity's workforce must be trained in PHI policies and procedures. New members must be trained within a reasonable period of time after joining the workforce. In addition, whenever material changes are made to policies and procedures regarding privacy, the workforce must receive additional training (Rinehart-Thompson 2017e, 256).

209. **b** Encryption is a technical method that reduces access and viewing of ePHI by unauthorized users. Encryption is defined as the process of transforming text into an unintelligible string of characters that can be transmitted via communications media with a high degree of security and then decrypted when it reaches a secure destination (Biedermann and Dolezel 2017, 394).

210. **d** One of the most significant changes under the Health Information Technology for Economic and Clinical Health Act (HITECH) is the increased inclusion and visibility of business associates (BAs). HIPAA regulations now apply to BAs for the first time, and this includes increased exposure to liability. In addition to expanding the scope of those who are BAs, even without a contract or BAA, HITECH now specifically includes the following as BAs: patient safety organizations (PSOs), which receive information in order to analyze patient safety issues; health information exchanges (HIEs) and health information organizations, which electronically share health information among providers; e-prescribing gateways, which serve as intermediaries between prescribing physicians and pharmacies; other persons who facilitate data transmissions; and personal health record (PHR) vendors that, by contract, enable covered entities to offer PHRs to their patients as part of the covered entity's electronic health record (ARRA 2009; AHIMA 2010; Rinehart-Thompson 2013, 147–148).

211. **c** Sometimes an individual's consent to a medical exam or intervention is not freely given, but is instead ordered by a court or through some other governmental action. This situation most often arises when the welfare of the public outweighs the individual's right to withhold consent (Klaver 2017b, 154–155).

212. **c** Access control requires the implementation of technical policies and procedures for electronic information systems that maintain electronic protected health information (ePHI) to allow access only to those persons or software programs that have been granted access rights as specified in the administrative safeguards. There are four implementation specifications with this standard, one of which includes emergency access procedures, which are procedures established to grant individuals access to ePHI in an emergency (Reynolds and Brodnik 2017a, 276–277).

213. **d** Access to information may be denied in some situations because it is specifically exempted from access by the Privacy Rule or it is not part of the designated record set. The Privacy Rule preamble makes clear that individuals do not have the right of access to psychotherapy notes (Rinehart-Thompson 2017d, 244).

214. **d** One of the biggest risk areas is the control of portable devices that contain ePHI. This area is particularly important because their use is growing and the likelihood of losing portable devices either accidentally or as the result of malicious acts is great. Portable devices include laptop and notebook computers, smartphones, CDs, personal digital assistants, USB drives, and handheld dictation devices. Data from the United States Department of Health and Human Services (HHS) shows that laptop theft is the most frequent cause of health information breaches, affecting 500 or more people (HHS 2012; Rinehart-Thompson 2013, 87–88).

215. **b** The release of information is a function of doing business and thus has a cost associated with it. The HIPAA Privacy Rule permits reasonable, cost-based charges for labor, postage, and supplies involved in photocopying health information for the patient and his or her personal representative (Brodnik 2017b, 372–373).

216. **a** Covered entities must establish who in their organization is responsible for compliance with the Security Rule requirements. This position is similar in scope to the privacy officer required by the HIPAA Privacy Rule. Covered entities may (but are not required to) appoint the same individual to fill the role of both the privacy and security officer (Biedermann and Dolezel 2017, 384).

217. **a** Data security management involves defending of safeguarding access to information. Only those individuals who need to know information should be authorized to access it (Johns 2016, 84).

218. **c** Administrative safeguards comprise over half of all the safeguards included in the Security Rule. Administrative safeguards are administrative actions such as policies, procedures, and documentation retention. These administrative safeguards are meant to manage the selection, development, implementation, and maintenance of security measures to protect ePHI and manage the conduct of the covered entities or business associates workforce (Biedermann and Dolezel 2017, 383).

219. **d** Humans are the most constant threat to health information integrity. Whether intentional or unintentional, incidents resulting from internal human threats are more common than incidents resulting from external human threats because individuals within an organization often have constant access to large amounts of information. Because intentional breaches are often committed by disgruntled employees, organizations should avoid offering employment with access to patient information to individuals who often change jobs (Rinehart-Thompson 2013, 118–119).

220. **c** A firewall is either a hardware or software device that examines traffic entering and leaving a network. It prevents some traffic from entering or leaving based on established rules. The term *firewall* can be used to describe the software that protects computing resources or to describe the combination of the software, hardware, and policies that protect the resources. The most common place to find a firewall is between the healthcare organization's internal network (trusted network) and the Internet (untrusted network). A firewall limits users on the Internet from accessing certain portions of the healthcare network and also limits internal users from accessing various portions of the Internet. As important as firewalls are to the overall security of health information systems, they cannot protect a system from all types of attacks (Sandefer 2016a, 366).

Domain 3

221. **d** X12N refers to standards adopted for electronic data interchange. In order for transmission of healthcare data between a provider and payer, both parties must adhere to these standards (Sayles and Trawick 2014, 175).

222. **a** Benchmarking is the systematic comparison of the products, services, and outcomes of an organization with those of a similar organization. Benchmarking comparisons also can be made using regional and national standards or some combination (Shaw and Carter 2015, 46).

223. **a** A check sheet is used to gather data on sample observations in order to detect patterns. When preparing to collect data, a team should consider the four W questions: Who will collect the data? What data will be collected? Where will the data be collected? When will the data be collected? Check sheets make it possible to systematically collect a large volume of data (Shaw and Carter 2015, 78–80).

224. **c** Reliability is frequently checked by having more than one person abstract data for the same case. The results are then compared to identify any discrepancies. This is called an interrater reliability method of checking. Several different people may be used to do the checking. In the cancer registry, physician members of the cancer committee are called on to check the reliability of the data (Forrestal 2016, 589).

225. **c** Although there are many different models of the SDLC, all generally include a variation of the following four phases: analysis, design, implementation, and maintenance and evaluation. Alignment and improvement are not included in the four phases of the SDLC (Amatayakul 2017, 46).

226. **d** Secondary analysis is the analysis of the original work of others. In secondary analysis, researchers reanalyze original data by combining data sets to answer new questions or by using more sophisticated statistical techniques. The work of others created the MEDPAR file (Forrestal 2016, 586).

227. **a** Clinical information systems (or applications) contain primarily clinical or health-related data that are used to diagnose, treat, monitor, and manage patient care. Examples of clinical applications include ancillary departmental systems (such as pharmacy, radiology, and laboratory medicine) as well as EMR systems, computerized provider order entry, medication administration, and nursing documentation (Sayles and Trawick 2014, 139–141).

228. **c** Because mandatory reporting of breaches was not required until YR-4, the number of breaches cannot be adequately estimated before that time, therefore, comparisons cannot be made between data before YR-4 and data after YR-4. Practitioners and other health professionals are faced with almost insurmountable amounts of data. This information is ultimately utilized for decision making. However, given the volume, variety, and complexity of the data, there is the potential for errors in decision making. Charts and graphs can help supplement human information processes to maximize the efficiency of interpreting data while minimizing interpretation errors (Marc 2016, 539–540).

229. **a** The prevalence rate is the proportion of persons in a population who have a particular disease at a specific point in time or over a specified period of time. The prevalence rate describes the magnitude of an epidemic and can be an indicator of the medical resources needed in a community for the duration of the epidemic (Edgerton 2016, 503).

230. **a** The Institutional Review Board (IRB) is a committee established to protect the rights and welfare of human research subjects involved in research activities. The IRB determines whether research is appropriate and protects human subjects as they participate in this research. The primary focus of the IRB is not on whether the type of research is appropriate for the organization to conduct but upon whether or not human subjects are adequately protected (Watzlaf 2016, 612).

231. **a** A survey is a common tool used in performance improvement to assess the level of satisfaction with a process by its customers. When designing a survey, the PI team must define the goal of the survey in clear and precise terms (Shaw and Carter 2015, 132–134).

232. **c** Control charts can be used to measure key processes over time. Using a control chart focuses attention on any variation in a process (Shaw and Carter 2015, 94).

233. **a** Case-mix index is the weighted average of the sum of the relative weights of all patients treated during a specified time period (Casto and Forrestal 2015, 115).

234. **c** Core (performance) measures are considered tools—standardized metrics—that provide an indication of an organization's performance. Core measures are defined as standardized sets of valid, reliable, and evidenced-based measures implemented by the Joint Commission (Shaw and Carter 2015, 18).

235. **a** The medical staff and the healthcare organization should work together to provide an environment that reduces the risk of infections in both patients and healthcare providers. The healthcare organization should support activities that look for, prevent, and control infections. An infection review is done with the involvement of the medical staff. Information is collected regularly on endemic and epidemic healthcare-associated infections. As appropriate, the healthcare organization must report significant information to both internal groups and public health agencies (Shaw and Carter 2015, 191).

236. **b** Strategic IS planning is the process of identifying and prioritizing IS needs based on the healthcare organization's mission and strategic goals (Amatayakul 2016, 389–390).

237. **a** The staffing level is determined by dividing the number of images by the expected productivity. An FTE is the total number of workers, including part-time, in an area as the equivalent of full-time positions. Divide 48,000 by maximum standard work per hour for each function then add up the calculated hours for each function and divide by 8 (Horton 2016, 186–187).

238. **b** Correlation is the statistic that is used to describe the association or relationship between two variables. In the healthcare setting, we may note that length of stay and charges are highly related or correlated (White 2016b, 526–527).

239. **a** Basic healthcare operations questions may often be analyzed using confidence intervals or hypothesis tests. A confidence interval is a range of values, such that the probability of that range covering the true value of a parameter is a set probability or confidence (White 2016b, 513).

240. **c** Personal health records electronically populate elements or subsets of protected health information (PHI) from provider organization databases into the electronic records of authorized patients, their families, other providers, and sometimes health payers and employers. A range of people and groups maintain the records, including the patients, their families, and other providers (Reynolds and Sharp 2016, 115–116).

241. **d** Skewness is the horizontal stretching of a frequency distribution to one side or the other so that one tail is longer than the other. The direction of skewness is on the side of the long tail. Thus, if the longer tail is on the right, the curve is skewed to the right. If the longer tail is on the left, the curve is skewed to the left (Horton 2016, 234).

242. **d** The range is the simplest measure of spread. It is the difference between the smallest and largest values in a frequency distribution:

$$\text{Range} = X_{max} - X_{min}$$

For this scenario, the range is 1 to 29 (29 – 1) or 28 (Horton 2016, 228).

243. **a** Predictive modeling applies statistical techniques to determine the likelihood of certain events occurring together (White 2013, 7).

244. **c** Simple linear regression (SLR) is another type of statistical inference that not only measures the strength of the relationship between two variables, but also estimates a functional relationship between them. SLR may be used when one of the two variables of interest is dependent on the other (White 2016b, 527–528).

245. **c** Hospital-acquired (nosocomial) infection rates may be calculated for the entire hospital or for a specific unit in the hospital. They also may be calculated for the specific types of infections. Ideally, the hospital should strive for an infection rate of 0.0 percent. The formula for calculating the hospital-acquired, or nosocomial, infection rate is: Total number of hospital-acquired infections for a given period / Total number of discharges, including deaths, for the same period × 100 (Edgerton 2016, 499).

246. **a** Auditing a random selection of EHR documentation would be the best approach for avoiding selection bias and in determining how the copy function is being used (Forrestal 2016, 593).

247. **b** A histogram is used to display a frequency distribution. It is different from a bar graph in that a bar graph is used to display data that fall into groups or categories (nominal or ordinal data) when the categories are noncontinuous or discrete (Marc 2016, 546).

248. **d** The master patient index (MPI) is a permanent database including every patient ever admitted to or treated by the facility. Even though patient health records may be destroyed after legal retention periods have been met, the information contained in the MPI must be kept permanently (Reynolds and Sharp 2016, 129).

249. **a** A use case analysis is a technique that describes an interaction between a user and a system. A use case diagram displays the relationship among actors and use cases. The two main components of a use case diagram are use cases and actors. An actor represents a user or another system that will interact with the system being modeled. A use case is an external view of the system that represents some action the user might perform in order to complete a task (Oachs 2016, 824–825).

250. **b** A bill cannot be generated until the coding is complete, so organizations routinely monitor the discharged, no final bill (DNFB) days. Generally this is done by reviewing the DNFB report that includes all patients who have been discharged from the facility, but for whom the billing process is not complete (Malmgren and Solberg 2016, 254–255).

251. **d** The estimated number of file shelves needed is based on several factors. One consideration is the average size of individual records. The volume of patients and the number of repeat visits or readmissions affect the potential expansion of each individual patient record. The type of facility also affects the size of individual records. For this equation, multiply anticipated discharges by projected number of years (2,000 × 10 years = 20,000). Because records average a 2-inch thickness, 40,000 filing inches are needed (20,000 × 2 = 40,000). Because each 5-shelf unit will have 165 linear filing inches available (33 × 5 = 165), the number of inches needed, 40,000, must be divided by 165 to determine the number of filing units that must be purchased, which will be 243 (242.4) (Reynolds and Sharp 2016, 133).

252. **d** Scatter diagrams are used to plot the points for two continuous variables that may be related to each other in some way. Whenever a scatter diagram indicates that the points are moving together in one direction or another, conclusions about the variables' relationship, either positive or negative, become evident. In this case a positive relationship between the variables can be seen as the points gather together at the top of the diagram (Oachs 2016, 816–817).

253. **c** The standard deviation (SD) is the square root of the variance. As such, it can be more easily interpreted as a measure of variation. If the SD is small, there is less dispersion around the mean. If the SD is large, there is greater dispersion around the mean (Horton 2016, 231).

254. **d** The term data analytics is used to describe a variety of approaches to using data to make business decisions. Healthcare data analytics is therefore the practice of using data to make business decisions in healthcare. More specifically, healthcare data analytics is the application of statistical techniques to allow informed decisions to be made based on the data (White 2016b, 510).

255. **a** A clinical data repository is a centralized database that captures, sorts, and processes patient data and then sends it back to the user (Russo 2013b, 322).

256. **a** A disease index is a listing in diagnosis code number order for patients discharged from the facility during a particular time period. Each patient's diagnoses are converted from a verbal description to a numerical code, usually using a coding system such as the International Classification of Diseases (ICD) (Sharp and Madlock-Brown 2016, 172).

257. **d** The focused review indicated areas of risk related to lower weighted MS-DRGs from triple and pair combinations which may be the result of a coder missing secondary diagnoses. A focused audit based on this specific potential problem area could help to identify these cases. Optimization seeks the most accurate documentation, coded data, and resulting payment in the amount the provider is rightly and legally entitled to receive (Hunt 2016, 286).

258. **b** The opposite of best-of-breed is best-of-fit. In this situation, virtually (though not absolutely) all applications are provided by a single vendor. This frequently makes it easier to add new applications from that vendor, but potentially even more difficult to add products from other vendors. Many organizations find their best-of-fit financial or administrative and operational system vendor is not as strong in EHR as they would desire. Alternatively, best-of-breed organizations find it difficult and costly to sustain this approach (Amatayakul 2017, 72–73).

259. **c** The hospital-acquired infection rate is $(4 \times 100) / 57 = 400 / 57 = 7.0\%$. Hospital-acquired (nosocomial) infection rates may be calculated for the entire hospital. They also may be calculated for the specific types of infections. Ideally, the hospital should strive for an infection rate of 0.0 percent (McCann 2016, 499).

260. **a** The use of CPOE can lead to significant improvements in patient safety because of the reminders or alerts built into the system. Although alerts and reminders are useful, too many become frustrating to the physicians because they have to constantly stop their data entry to address the alerts and reminders (Sayles and Trawick 2014, 162).

261. **c** During the implementation phase of the SDLC, a comprehensive plan for implementing the new system is developed. This plan would include all plans for training managers, technical staff, and other end-users (Amatayakul 2017, 46).

262. **a** During the analysis phase, the need for a new information system is explored further, problems with the existing system are solidified, and user needs are identified (Amatayakul 2017, 46).

263. **a** Hospital Consumer Assessment of Healthcare Providers (HCAHPS) is standardized assessment of consumer perspectives regarding healthcare access and quality (CAHPS) by the Centers for Medicaid and Medicare Services (CMS Systems (HCAHPS) (Sandefer 2016b, 426).

264. **c** Under the inpatient rehabilitation facility PPS (IRF-PPS) system, each patient is assigned to a case-mix group (CMG) and a tier within the CMG. The CMG assignment is based on the primary condition for which the patient was admitted to the IRF or inpatient unit and on the patient's functional and cognitive abilities at the time of the admission. The tier assignment is based on the presence of one or more specified secondary diagnoses, or comorbidities, that affect the resources needed to treat the patient. Each CMG and tier is assigned a relative weight (RW) that serves as the basis for the payment rate. The payment rate is adjusted at the facility level for teaching status, the applicable geographic wage index, and the percentage of low-income patients served by the facility. Cases with extraordinarily high costs compared to the prospectively set payment may qualify for an outlier payment (Hazelwood and Venable 2016, 223, 225).

265. **b** The federated architectural type has become more prevalent for health information organizations. There are two forms of this architecture. The consistent federated form is very similar to the consolidated architecture in which the data repository is partitioned but centrally managed. The consistent federated form, however, takes this one step further and physically separates the data but still offers centralized management. Essentially, this is much like an application service provider (ASP) or software as a service (SaaS) model of acquiring software (Amatayakul 2017, 417–418).

266. **c** The median is the midpoint of a frequency distribution and falls in the ordinal scale of measurement. It is the point at which 50 percent of the observations fall above and 50 percent fall below. If an odd number of observations is in the frequency distribution, the median is the middle number. In this data set, 8 is the middle number (Horton 2016, 222).

267. **d** The proportionate mortality ratio (PMR) is a measure of mortality due to a specific cause for a specific time period. In the formula for calculating the PMR, the numerator is the number of deaths due to a specific disease for a specific time period, and the denominator is the number of deaths from all causes for the same time period. The proportionate mortality ratio for diabetes mellitus = 73,249 / 2,443,387 = 0.03 × 100 = 3.0% (AHIMA 2014, 121; Edgerton 2016, 484–485).

268. **c** The master patient index (MPI) is a database that maintains a unique identifier for each patient seen at the organizational or enterprise level. Correctly identifying the elements of the MPI is very important. The MPI, whether in paper or electronic format, is the most important resource in a healthcare facility because it tracks patient activity across every type of healthcare setting (Fahrenholz 2013c, 155).

269. **b** Because there is no mandated unique patient identifier, ensuring that the HIE organization can identify the right patient as it seeks to exchange information is a process of identity matching (Amatayakul 2017, 419).

270. **d** Unstructured clinical information would include notes written by the physicians and other practitioners who treat the patient, dictated and transcribed reports, and legal forms such as consents and advanced directives to name a few (Biedermann and Dolezel 2017, 84).

271. **b** Health informatics must consider the development of standards for software to be used in the EHR and the exchange of data. Compatibility and interoperability, allowing different health information systems to work together within and across organizational boundaries in order to advance the effective delivery of healthcare for individuals and communities, are a key focus in health informatics (Biedermann and Dolezel 2017, 22).

272. **b** Regional Extension Centers were created with the purpose of providing needed support for physicians in selecting, implementing, and utilizing systems to further the deployment of EHR systems in their practices (Biedermann and Dolezel 2017, 79–80).

273. **a** Best-of-breed is when an organization has acquired the "best" products from various vendors. The result is that each individual organizational unit may be happy with its chosen product, but as the organization moves toward adding clinical components that rely on the various other systems as a source of data or to which data must be sent, the challenge to exchange such data can be overwhelming (Amatayakul 2017, 72–73).

274. **d** Straight turnover refers to having everyone in the designated group go live at one time, with paper processes ceasing virtually immediately after go-live. This is the most typical form of turnover for EHRs because most organizations find that any reliance on former paper processing not only ends up being too time-consuming but also sends a message that the system is not to be trusted (Amatayakul 2017, 254).

275. **c** Within healthcare, standard protocols that support communication between nonintegrated applications are often referred to as messaging standards, also called interoperability standards or data exchange standards. Messaging standards provide the tools to map proprietary formats to one another and more easily accomplish the exchange of data (Amatayakul 2017, 400–401).

276. **c** For whatever architecture an HIE organization may have, there needs to be a way to identify participants, which may include individual providers, representatives of payer organizations, and patients or consumers, as well as organizational entities and their information systems. This service is called registry and directory (Amatayakul 2017, 418–419).

277. **c** The median offers the following three advantages: relatively easy to calculate; based on the whole distribution and not just a portion of it, as is the case with the mode; and unlike the mean, it is not influenced by extreme values or unusual outliers in the frequency distribution (Horton 2016, 222).

278. **a** As facilities transition from paper-based health records to EHRs, the often lengthy transition forces healthcare facilities to manage and maintain hybrid health records. A hybrid health record is a system with functional components that includes both paper and electronic documents and uses both manual and electronic components (Russo 2013b, 334).

279. **d** Physiological signal processing systems, such as ECG, EEG, and FHR tracing systems, store data based on the body's signals and create output based on the lines plotted between the signals' points. The data type used by these systems is referred to as signal tracing or vector graphic data (Sandefer 2016a, 358).

280. **b** In data mining, the analyst performs exploratory data analysis to determine trends and identify patterns in the data set. Data mining is sometimes referred to as knowledge discovery (White 2016b, 531).

281. **a** In 2016 the EHR Incentive Program for physician and individual providers was discontinued as a separate program. The use of EHRs will be combined with quality measures and other items in payment and penalty consideration under the Medicare program (Biedermann and Dolezel 2017, 95).

282. **c** A secure patient portal does allow for the communication between the provider and the patient and is not just a site for patients to access information. This is part of the effort to engage patients in their care (Biedermann and Dolezel 2017, 458).

283. **a** Parallel processing is a turnover strategy where the organization continues processing in manual form as well as electronic form. The intent is to validate the electronic processing against the manual processing (Amatayakul 2017, 254).

284. **b** During the implementation phase of the SDLC, a comprehensive plan for implementing the new system is developed. This plan would include all plans for training managers, technical staff, and other end-users (Amatayakul 2017, 46).

285. **b** Mainframe computers use a single large computer with many terminals directly connected to it and sharing the resources of the single computer (Amatayakul 2017, 333).

286. **a** When developing the data elements that go into a database, the fields should be normalized. Normalization is breaking the data elements into the level of detail desired by the facility. For example, last name and first name should be in separate fields as should city, state, and zip code (Sayles and Trawick 2014, 51).

287. **a** Health record storage is the application of efficient procedures for the use of filing equipment and storage media to keep records secure and available to those providers and other healthcare personnel authorized to access them (Reynolds and Sharp 2016, 131).

288. **d** An interface is software that works between two or more systems to enable the two systems to share data (Amatayakul 2016, 402).

289. **d** Many hospitals incorporate documents into their EHR systems using image-processing technology. A digital scanner creates images of handwritten and printed documents that are then stored in health record databases as electronic files. Using scanned images solves many of the problems associated with traditional paper-based health records (Russo 2013b, 335).

290. **d** Data about patients can be extracted from individual health records and combined as aggregate data. Aggregate data are used to develop information about groups of patients. In this case, the fact that 50 percent of patients treated at our facilities have Medicare as their primary payer is data about patients combined together, so it is aggregate data (Sharp and Madlock-Brown 2016, 170).

291. **d** The probability of making a Type I error based on a particular set of data is called the p-value (White 2016b, 514).

292. **b** To enhance retrieval of scanned documents, some form of indexing needs to take place in order to organize the documents. Ideally, each form that is scanned or otherwise created should have a bar code or some other forms recognition feature, or features, associated with it (Amatayakul 2017, 285).

293. **c** Bus topology is the simplest network topology, connecting one device to another along a "backbone". A major disadvantage is that the central cable is a single point of failure. If this cable fails for any reason then the entire network goes down (Johns 2015, 57).

294. **a** One benefit of the unit numbering system is that all records for a specific patient, both inpatient and outpatient, are kept together (Reynolds and Sharp 2016, 128).

295. **c** If the sample has extreme values on either the high or low end of the scale, then the median may be the better choice for describing the center of the distribution. The median is less influenced by outliers (White 2016b, 520).

296. **a** Client or server architecture is the predominant form of computer architecture used in healthcare associations today. In client/server architecture, certain computers (servers) have been configured to perform most of the processing and resource-intensive tasks, while other computers (clients), which generally are less-powerful computers, capture, view, and perform limited processes on data (Amatayakul 2017, 333–334).

297. **c** The capability to retrieve documents from an electronic document management system (EDMS) is determined by the underlying technology used to store the documents. In addition to bar codes on medical record documents, optical character recognition (OCR) may be available to enhance the accuracy of indexing features on forms (Sandefer 2016a, 352).

298. **d** Firewalls, encryption, and biometrics are technologies used to enable security in healthcare information systems. Telemedicine is not a technology used to enable security (Sandefer 2016a, 365–366).

299. **b** Structured query language (SQL) includes both data dictionary language and data manipulation language components and is used to create and manipulate relational databases (Sayles and Trawick 2014, 107).

300. **a** A benefits realization study is an evaluation of the financial benefits that have accrued from the investment made in the project . It may be performed at specific milestones in the life of the project and used to help in future systems planning, designing, and implementing (Amatayakul 2017, 106).

301. **c** Contingency and disaster planning prepare the facility to operate in a manual process and to get the information systems up and operational again. When the systems are again functional, data recovery must occur. Data captured during the downtime must be entered into the system in order to bring the system up-to-date. Data lost out of the database should be recoverable from backup tapes or other media. Depending on the time since the last backup, little or no data may be lost (Sayles and Trawick 2014, 213).

302. **b** E-health is the application of e-commerce to the healthcare industry. These include the links among the healthcare trading and business partners; the links to healthcare equipment and supply vendors, providers, and health plans; and the transactions for exchanging data on healthcare eligibility, referrals, claims, and so forth. Bedside nursing care, direct patient care, and emergency room records are all EHR applications and therefore not e-health applications (Sandefer 2016a, 354).

303. **a** Unit numbering storage is a health record identification system in which the patient receives a unique medical record number at the time of the first encounter that is used for all subsequent encounters (Reynolds and Sharp 2016, 128).

304. **d** A web portal is a single point of personalized access (an entryway) through which to find and deliver information (content), applications, and services. Web portals began in the consumer market as an integration strategy rather than a solution. Portals offered users of the large, public Internet service provider websites, fast, centralized access (via a web browser) to an array of Internet services and information found on those websites (Sandefer 2016a, 355).

305. **c** Enterprise master patient indexes (EMPIs) provide access to multiple repositories of information from overlapping patient populations that are maintained in separate systems and databases. This occurs through an indexing scheme to all unique patient identification numbers and information in all the organizations' databases. As such, EMPIs become the cornerstones of healthcare system integration projects (Reynolds and Sharp 2016, 129–131).

306. **a** Star topology is one physical topology of a network and uses a central hub that connects all of the data on the network. All data has to pass through the hub which then forwards it to its correct destination (Johns 2015, 57).

307. **a** If an EHR is to provide clinical decision support it requires two things: structured data and a clinical data repository (Sandefer 2016a, 364).

308. **a** Preventive controls are front-end processes that guide work in such a way that input and process variations are minimized. Simple things such as standard operating procedures, edits on data entered into computer-based systems, and training processes are ways to reduce the potential for error by using preventive controls (Oachs 2016, 804).

309. **c** A data flow diagram is a diagram of how data flows in the database. The data flow diagram is a good way to show management and other nontechnical users the system design (Sayles and Trawick 2014, 56).

310. **a** Typically, provider-based portals uses include requesting prescription renewal, scheduling appointments, and asking questions of providers via secure messaging. Patients may also pay bills online or securely view all or portions of the electronic health record, such as current medical conditions, medications, allergies, and test results. Patients would not be able to edit their health record information (Sandefer 2016a, 355).

311. **d** Statistical techniques are used in predictive modeling to create a model to assess the likelihood or probability of fraudulent claims. These statistical techniques include logistical regression, cluster analysis, or decision trees. A data warehouse is not a statistical technique that would be used for this purpose (White 2016b, 532).

312. **d** The HIE's record locator service (RLS) manages the pointers to the information on the servers of the HIE participants. The pointers in a RLS can include a person identification number (person ID) and metadata. The RLS does not provide information about the record, it merely points to where it might be found. Data are not stored in a centralized database and records are only provided when queried (McCann 2016, 454).

313. **b** Big bang roll out is the implementation of all aspects of the EHR component (or entire EHR in an ambulatory setting) in all organizational units virtually simultaneously (Amatayakul 2017, 253).

314. **d** In a terminal-digit filing system, records are filed according to a three-part number made up of two-digit pairs. The basic terminal-digit filing system contains 10,000 divisions, made up of 100 sections ranging from 00 to 99 with 100 divisions within each section ranging from 00 to 99. In a terminal-digit filing system, the shelving units (filing space) are equally divided into 100 sections (Reynolds and Sharp 2016, 128–129).

315. **c** Health Level 7 (HL7) is a nonprofit organization that develops standards for interoperability of health information technology (Fahrenholz 2013a, 44).

316. **a** Extranets are networks that connect a given organization to its customers and business partners or suppliers (business associates in healthcare). Although extranets send information over public networks, requiring a greater level of security, access to them is still restricted to the services and persons authorized (Sandefer 2016a, 356).

317. **c** The Joint Commission specifies that the number of delinquent records cannot exceed 50 percent of the average number of discharges (Reynolds and Sharp 2016, 126).

318. **c** Algorithms are mathematical formulas used by an organization or enterprise that combine weighted data elements to determine the probability of a duplicate in order identify potential duplicate master patient index (MPI) entries. There are three types of matching algorithms available in the industry today: deterministic, rules based, and probabilistic. The matching algorithm is a critical component of any successful MPI solution (Fahrenholz 2013, 169).

319. **d** Controls for accuracy of the MPI include limiting access to the index and limiting the ability to make changes to a few key personnel. The first step to maintaining an accurate index is to obtain the correct information at admission or registration (Reynolds and Sharp 2016, 130).

320. **b** Consumer health informatics is a field devoted to informatics from multiple consumer or patient views and includes patient-focused informatics, health literacy, and consumer education, with a focus on information structures and processes that empower consumers to manage their own health (AMIA 2015; Sandefer 2016b, 425).

321. **b** The first step in statistical hypothesis testing is defining the null and alternative hypotheses. The null hypothesis is the status quo. In this example the readmission rates are equal would be the null hypothesis showing no relationship between the two hospitals (White 2016a, 65).

322. **c** A master patient index (MPI) is an index of known patients within a single organization whose visits are linked together by a single identifier, typically the medical records number. Some recommended core data elements for the MPI are: name, address, gender, date of birth, and many others. Accession number, revenue code, and charge code are not recommended core data elements for the MPI (Fahrenholz 2013c, 176–178).

323. **b** LOINC is a well-accepted set of terminology standards that provide a standard set of universal names and codes for identifying individual laboratory and clinical results (Palkie 2016a, 155).

324. **b** The contingency plan standard is central to being able to ensure availability of data. The standard requires covered entities to establish and implement as-needed policies and procedures for responding to an emergency or other occurrence. These policies and procedures include a data back up plan, disaster recovery plan, and emergency mode operation plan. An environmental risk plan is not part of the implementation specification (Biedermann and Dolezel 2017, 387).

325. **b** In data mining, the analyst performs exploratory data analysis to determine trends and identify patterns in the data set (White 2016b, 531).

326. **d** The Digital Imaging and Communications in Medicine (DICOM) standard supports retrieval of information from imaging devices and equipment to diagnostic and review workstations as well as short-term and long-term storage systems (Amatayakul 2017, 404–405).

327. **b** The alternative hypothesis is the compliment of the null hypothesis and typically requires some action to be taken. In this scenario, the analyst is comparing emergency department wait times between weekends and weekdays. The alternative hypothesis would be that the average wait time is longer on weekends (White 2016a, 65).

328. **d** A scatter diagram is a data analysis tool used to plot points of two variables suspected of being related to each other in some way (Oachs 2016, 816–817).

329. **a** MPI management must include continuous maintenance and correction of data integrity problems. Ongoing education of registration and scheduling staff is critical to maintaining low creation rates for duplicates, overlays, and other EMPI data integrity problems (Reynolds and Sharp 2016, 130).

330. **c** The centralized HIE model stores patient records in a single database built to allow queries into the system. This model tends to return results quicker than other models. The ownership of the data is a difficult question to settle between all participants, as is how to ensure the accuracy of the data (McCann 2016, 454).

331. **b** To calculate the case mix index from the volume of cases from MS-DRG calculate the weighted average MS-DRG weight by completing these steps: (1) Multiply the number of discharges in each MS-DRG by the relative weight of that MS-DRG; (2) Sum the relative weights from step 1; (3) Sum the number of discharges in the MS-DRGs chosen to be evaluated; (4) Divide the total relative weights from step 2 by the total number of discharges from step 3.

Step 1:

$3.6918 \times 100 = 369.18$

$2.1965 \times 52 = 114.218$

$1.6610 \times 36 = 59.796$

Step 2:

$369.18 + 114.218 + 59.796 = 543.194$

Step 3:

100 + 52 + 36 = 188

Step 4:

543.194 / 188 = **2.8893**

(White 2016a, 155–156)

Domain 4

332. **d** The process for adding a new technology into the charge description master (CDM) includes reviewing new technology for FDA approval, for OPPS pass-through assignment, and also to have a coding professional check the codes from the manufacturer for accuracy (Schraffenberger and Kuehn, 2011, 234).

333. **c** Resolving failed edits is one of many duties of the health information management (HIM) department. Various medical departments depend on the coding expertise of HIM professionals to avoid incorrect coding and potential compliance issues (Schraffenberger and Kuehn 2011, 237–238).

334. **a** A bill cannot be generated until the coding is complete, so organizations routinely monitor the discharged, no final bill (DNFB) days. Generally this is done by reviewing the DNFB report that includes all patients who have been discharged from the facility, but for whom the billing process is not complete (Malmgren and Solberg 2016, 254–255).

335. **d** The Integrated Outpatient Code Editor (IOCE) is a predefined set of edits created by Medicare to check outpatient claims for compliance with the Medicare outpatient prospective payment system (OPPS). The IOCE will review a coded claim for accuracy and send back an edit flag if an error has been detected in the claim. Most organizations run all their claims through the IOCE prior to sending out to any payer to look for errors, correct them, and then send out a clean claim. A portion of the NCCI edits are embedded in the IOCE edits (Schraffenberger and Kuehn 2011, 465).

336. **c** Each Resource-Based Relative Value Scale (RBRVS) comprises three elements: physician work, physician practice expense, and malpractice, each of which is a national average available in the *Federal Register* (Casto and Forrestal 2015, 150).

337. **a** A query is routine communication and education tool used to advocate for complete and compliant documentation. The intent is to clarify what has been recorded, not to call into question the provider's clinical judgment or medical expertise. This is an example of a circumstance where the chronic condition must be verified. All secondary conditions must match the definition in the UHDDS and whether the COPD does is not clear (Hunt 2016, 276–277).

338. **d** Coverage not in effect for date of service is not a most common reason for claims denials as effective dates of coverage are usually resolved in the front end of the revenue cycle or prior to submission of the bill to payers (Malmgren and Solberg 2016, 243).

339. **a** Nonparticipating providers (nonPARs) do not sign a participation agreement with Medicare but may or may not accept assignment. If the nonPAR physician elects to accept assignment, he or she is paid 95 percent (5 percent less than participating physicians) of the Medicare fee schedule (MFS). For example, if the MFS amount is $200, the PAR provider receives $160 (80 percent of $200), but the nonPAR provider receives only $152 (95 percent of $160). In this case the physician is nonparticipating so he or she will receive 95 percent of the 80 percent of the MFS or 80 percent of 300, which is $240; 95 percent of the $240 is $228 (Casto and Forrestal 2015, 153–154).

340. **c** Often the consultant's report will identify specific issues or causes of coding variances that require further action. These items may include issuing queries to certain physicians to obtain additional information to modify the original coding, resubmitting claims to payers because the coding has been modified, discussing documentation deficiencies with one or more clinicians, addressing legibility issues with one or more physicians, and providing focused education to one or more coders. Another common error found includes duplicate codes (one from the coder assignment, also known as soft coding, and one from the CDM, also known as hard coding). This occurrence could cause duplicate payments by a payer and expose the organization to false billing allegations (Schraffenberger and Kuehn 2011, 324, 327).

341. **a** Long-term care hospitals (LTCHs) must meet state requirements for acute care hospitals and must have a provider agreement with Medicare in order to receive Medicare payments. Fiscal intermediaries verify that the LTCH meets the required average LOS of greater than 25 days (James 2013a, 514).

342. **b** Universal protocol incorporates the principles of eliminating wrong-site, wrong-procedure, and wrong-person surgery. The steps involved in this protocol include preoperative verification process, marking of the operative site, and a "time-out" before starting any procedure (Shaw and Carter 2015, 174–176).

343. **a** The policy information provided states this is a single policy or employee-only policy, so the member's spouse is not covered (Casto and Forrestal 2015, 58–59).

344. **b** The insured is the organization that has purchased the insurance policy. In this case, STATE has purchased the insurance coverage for subscriber Jane B. White (Casto and Forrestal 2015, 58–59).

345. **a** Hospitals must have a policy that establishes a time frame for completing the history and physical. Most facilities set the time frame as within the first 24 hours following admission and require that the history and physical be completed by the provider who is admitting the patient. CMS requires that the history and physical examination must be completed no more than 30 days before or 24 hours after admission and the report must be placed in the record within 24 hours after admission (Reynolds and Sharp 2016, 107–108).

346. **d** A CDI program provides a mechanism for the coding staff to communicate with the physician regarding nonspecific diagnostic statements or when additional diagnoses are suspected but not clearly stated in the record, which helps to avoid assumption coding (Hess 2015, 42).

347. **b** Every state has certain licensure regulations that healthcare facilities must meet in order to remain in operation. Licensure regulations may include very specific requirements (Fuller 2016, 31).

348. **a** When coders "optimize" the coding process, they attempt to make coding for reimbursement as accurate as possible. In this way, the healthcare facility can obtain the highest dollar amount justified within the terms of the government program or the insurance policy involved (Hunt 2016, 286).

349. **a** Medical identity theft can be the result of either internal or external forces. Electronic health records have improved the ability to share information, but this has also increased exposure to data making it more vulnerable. Internal medical identity theft is committed by organization insiders, such as clinical or administrative staff with access to patient information. External threats are causing a greater risk for healthcare organizations due to increased threats of ransomware, malware, and denial-of-service (DOS) attacks (Olenik and Reynolds 2017, 290).

350. **a** The conversion factor is an across-the-board multiplier that sets the allowance for the relative values—a constant (Casto and Forrestal 2015, 152).

351. **c** The formulary is composed of medications used for commonly occurring conditions or diagnoses treated in the healthcare organization. Organizations accredited by the Joint Commission are required to maintain a formulary and document that they review at least annually for a medication's continued safety and efficacy (Shaw and Carter 2015, 246).

352. **d** If a service is hard-coded into the charge description master (CDM), it is important that this decision is communicated to the coding staff. If the decision is not effectively communicated, the result could be duplicate billing that in turn could result in overpayment to the facility (Casto and Forrestal 2015, 253).

353. **c** Part of a coding compliance plan is to identify areas of risk through audits and monitoring. Selecting the types of cases to review is also important. Examples of various case selection possibilities include medical and surgical MS-DRSs by high dollar and volume. Auditing cases with infrequent diagnosis and procedure codes, low dollar and low volume, and low admission diagnoses would not be as suitable (Hunt 2016, 286).

354. **c** Under the home health prospective payment system (HHPPS), CMS has accounted for nonroutine medical supplies, home health aide visits, medical social services, and nursing and therapy services (Casto and Forrestal 2015, 235).

355. **d** Unbundling occurs when individual components of a complete procedure or service are billed separately instead of using a combination code (Bowman 2017, 440).

356. **c** Because clinical documentation improvement (CDI) involves the medical and clinical staffs, it is more likely that the CDI project will be successful if these staff are included in developing the process for documentation improvement. Because all hospital staff do not document in the health record, a memorandum from the CEO to all staff would not be efficient or necessarily effective. The chairperson of the CDI project does not have line authority for employee evaluation. The Joint Commission performs oversight activities but would not be involved in direct operational tasks such as this (Schraffenberger and Kuehn 2011, 360).

357. **c** In this example, DNFB met the benchmark in January, February, and June, which is 3/6 or 50 percent of the time (Malmgren and Solberg 2016, 254–255).

358. **c** When an organization has delivered goods or services, payment for the same is expected. Because the revenue has been accrued upon delivery or provision of the goods and services, the organization must have some way to keep track of what is owed to them as a result. Accounts receivable then is merely a list of the amounts due from various customers (in this case, patients). Payment on the individual amounts is expected within a specified period. A schedule of those expected amounts is prepared in order to track and follow up on payments that are overdue (late) (Revoir and Davis 2016, 840).

359. **c** Typical performance statistics maintained by the accounts receivable department include days in accounts receivable and aging of accounts. Aging of accounts is maintained in 30-day increments (0–30 days, 31–60 days, and so forth) (Casto and Forrestal 2015, 255).

360. **c** Managers and directors must be diligent at auditing and monitoring compliance in the coding unit. Reviewing and auditing through internal audits enables managers and directors to see coding issues firsthand. Education is needed to ensure that coding remains compliant. The director should review the errors and determine if the coding manager is not compliant with coding guidelines. If the manager is not compliant, the director needs to discuss the issues and counsel the employee in order to ensure coding guidelines are followed by all coding staff. (Casto and Forrestal 2015, 44–45).

361. **a** To meet the CMS's definition of an IRF, facilities must have an inpatient population in which at least 60 percent of the patients require intensive rehabilitation services and one of the 13 conditions: stroke, spinal cord injury, congenital deformity, amputation, major multiple trauma, fracture of femur, brain injury, neurological disorders, burns, active polyarticular rheumatoid arthritis, systemic vasculitides, severe or advanced osteo-arthritis, or knee or hip replacement (Casto and Forrestal 2015, 222–223).

362. **d** Coverage differs among these states because Medicaid allows states to maintain a unique program adapted to state residents' needs and average incomes. Although state programs must meet coverage requirements for groups such as recipients of adoption assistance and foster care, other types of coverage, such as vision and dental services, are determined by the states' Medicaid agencies (Casto and Forrestal 2015, 87).

363. **a** Healthcare entities should consider a policy in which queries may be appropriate when documentation in the patient record fails to meet one of the following five criteria: legibility, completeness, clarity, consistency, and precision (Hunt 2016, 276–277).

364. **a** Deemed status means accrediting bodies such as the Joint Commission or American Osteopathic Association can survey facilities for compliance with the Medicare Conditions of Participation for hospitals instead of government (James 2013a, 447).

365. **d** Under the Medicare hospital outpatient prospective payment system (OPPS), outpatient services such as recovery room, supplies (other than pass-through), and anesthesia are included in this reimbursement method (Casto and Forrestal 2015, 169).

366. **b** Both the MS-LTC-DRGs and the acute care MS-DRGs are based on the principal diagnosis in terms of grouping and reimbursement (Casto and Forrestal 2015, 217–218).

367. **b** The charge description master contains elements such as department and item number, item description, revenue code, HCPCS code, price, and activity status (Casto and Forrestal 2015, 257–262).

368. **a** In the claims reconciliation process, the healthcare facility uses the explanation of benefits, Medicare Summary Notice, and the remittance advice to reconcile accounts (Casto and Forrestal 2015, 256–257).

369. **a** Facilities may design a clinical documentation improvement (CDI) program based on several different models. Improvement work can be done with retrospective record review and queries, with concurrent record review and queries, or with concurrent coding. Although much of the CDI process is often done while the patient is in-house, it does not eliminate the need for post-discharge queries (Schraffenberger and Kuehn, 2011, 363).

370. **d** The last component of the revenue cycle is reconciliation and collections. The healthcare facility uses the explanation of benefits (EOB), Medicare summary notice (MSN), and remittance advice (RA) to reconcile accounts. EOBs and MSNs identify the amount owed by the patient to the facility. Collections can contact the patient to collect outstanding deductibles and copayments. RAs indicate rejected or denied items or claims. Facilities can review the RAs and determine where the claim error can be corrected and resubmitted for additional payment (Casto and Forrestal 2015, 256–257).

371. **c** The on-site Joint Commission survey utilizes a tracer methodology that permits assessment of operational systems and processes in relation to the actual experiences of selected patients currently under the organization's care. Patients are selected on the basis of the current census of patients that the organization identifies as typical of its case mix. As cases are examined in relation to the actual care processes, the surveyor may identify performance issues or trends in one or more steps of the process or in the interfaces between processes. Patients on subsequent days may be selected on the basis of issues raised (Shaw and Carter 2015, 412–413).

372. **d** The primary operational components of the CDI program are the record review and the query process. The review process and the physician query process allow for the highest level of quality in clinical documentation (Hess 2015, 158).

373. **b** The purpose of the recovery audit contractors (RAC) program is to reduce improper Medicare payments and prevent future improper payments made of claims of healthcare services to Medicare beneficiaries. Improper payments may be overpayments or underpayments (James 2013b, 453).

374. **d** Denials may simply be defined as a payer's refusal to provide payment. Approximately 90 percent of denials are preventable and 67 percent are recoverable. Some common reasons for denials include: billing noncovered services, lack of medical necessity, and beneficiary not covered. Coverage not in effect for the date of service is not a common reason for denial (Malmgren and Solberg 2016, 257).

375. **c** The charge description master can provide a method for grouping items that are frequently reported together. Items that must be reported separately but are used together, such as interventional radiology imaging and injection procedures, are called exploding charges (Schraffenberger and Kuehn 2011, 227).

376. **b** Like any organization, the medical staff, as a self-governing entity, needs to have structure. The medical staff bylaws provide an organizational structure to ensure communication with the governing body and high-quality patient care. Committees are used to help most medical staffs function. This committee structure is used to make credentialing and clinical privilege decisions (Reynolds and Brodnik 2017b, 476–478).

377. **a** The HIM department can plan focused reviews based on specific problem areas after the initial baseline review has been completed. This would be called a focused inpatient review (Schraffenberger and Kuehn 2011, 314–315).

378. **d** The Federal Trade Commission has oversight responsibility for identity theft regulations and requires financial institutions and creditors to develop and implement written identity theft prevention programs (Biederman and Dolezel 2017, 406).).

379. **c** In many instances, patients have more than one insurance policy and the determination of which policy is primary and which is secondary is necessary so that there is no duplication in payment of benefits. This process is called coordination of benefits (COB) (Casto and Forrestal 2015, 66).

380. **a** Hospitals should take the opportunity to review old Program for Evaluation Payment Patterns Electronic Reports (PEPPERs) to identify those claims that could be targeted by the recovery audit contractors (RACs). During the demonstration program in South Carolina, some hospitals were able to see a direct correlation of the DRGs and one day stays reviewed by the RAC in their PEPPER data. For example, one day stays for chest pain—DRG 143—were found to be an improper medical necessity error under the RAC, and comparison data in the PEPPER also showed this trend. PEPPERs can be a great tool for RAC preparation because they outline the hospital's Medicare payment patterns compared to other hospitals in the state (Wilson 2010, 29–30).

381. **a** An outlier payment is paid when the cost of the service is greater than the ambulatory payment classification (APC) payment by a fixed ratio and exceeds the APC payment plus a threshold amount (Casto and Forrestal 2015, 175).

382. **c** Answer c is the only option that provides a consistent and reliable method to improve communication and documentation. Options a and b do not provide any communication avenues that will improve documentation or provide coders with necessary information to assign accurate codes. Option d is not appropriate in any case because coders should not be making clinical judgments (Hunt 2016, 278–279).

383. **b** The HIM department can plan focused reviews based on specific problem areas after the initial baseline review has been completed. This would be called a focused inpatient review (Schraffenberger and Kuehn 2011, 314–315).

384. **b** The coder assigned the correct diagnosis code. The coder did not assign the correct procedure because the root operation for this procedure is reposition, not supplement. Reposition is moving to its normal location or other suitable location all or a portion of a body part, whereas supplement is defined as putting in or on biological or synthetic material that physically reinforces or augments the function of the portion of a body part (Kuehn and Jorwic 2017, 105–106).

385. **b** For Medicare patients, the fiscal intermediary and carriers prepare Medicare summary notices or MSNs. The MSN details amounts billed by the provider, amounts approved by Medicare, how much Medicare reimbursed the provider, and what the patient must pay the provider by way of deductible and copayments (Casto and Forrestal 2015, 256).

386. **a** The Joint Commission requires accredited hospitals and other healthcare facilities to implement systems for identifying and addressing sentinel events. A sentinel event is described as an unexpected occurrence involving death or serious physical or psychological injury, or the risk thereof (James 2013b, 467–468, 490).

387. **b** Ongoing evaluation is critical to successful coding and billing for third-party payer reimbursement. The goal of internal auditing is to protect providers from sanctions or fines (Palkie 2016b, 297–298).

388. **c** The length of multiple laceration repairs located in the same classification are added together and one code is assigned (Kuehn 2017, 110).

389. **c** In 2007, Identity Theft Red Flags and Address Discrepancy Rules were enacted as part of the Federal Fair and Accurate Credit Transactions Act (FATCA) of 2003. The FATCA requires financial institutions and creditors to develop and implement written identity theft programs that identify, detect, and respond to red flags that may signal the presence of identity theft (Olenik and Reynolds 2017, 291).

390. **b** As a result of the disparity in documentation practices by providers, querying has become a common communication and educational method to advocate proper documentation practices. Queries can be made in situations when there is clinical evidence for a higher degree of specificity or severity. In this situation the reason for the mechanical ventilation and intubation, most likely, is respiratory failure and the physician would need to be queried for validation of that diagnosis in order for it to be coded (Hunt 2016, 276–277).

391. **b** As healthcare organizations throughout the country have become more computer savvy, so too has the federal government. The data-mining efforts of the recovery audit contractors (RACs) allow them to deny payments without ever reviewing a health record. For example, duplicate billing, such as billing for two colonoscopies on the same day for the same Medicare beneficiary, is easy to identify as a potential improper payment. Through the use of the RACs' proprietary software, RACs are able to detect improper payments. Underpayment and overpayment amounts can be subject to an automated review (Wilson 2010, 15–16).

392. **c** The principal diagnosis is governed by the circumstances of admission, which in this case is dehydration (Schraffenberger and Palkie 2017, 140).

393. **a** Beneficiary incentive programs encourage Medicare beneficiaries to review their bills for discrepancies. QIO reviews can be prompted by a Medicare beneficiary through a complaint or a request for appeal, by federal agencies, or as a routine review of care and billing patterns under the Medicare program. All of these functions are referred to as "case review" (Wilson 2010, 12).

394. **d** Facilities may design a clinical documentation improvement (CDI) program based on several different models. Improvement work can be done with retrospective record review and queries, with concurrent record review and queries, or with concurrent coding. Although much of the CDI process is often done while the patient is in-house, it does not eliminate the need for post-discharge queries (Hunt 2016, 266).

Domain 5

395. **b** Alternate work schedules are alternatives to the regular 40-hour workweek; the following are examples: compressed workweek, flextime, and job sharing (Oachs 2016, 795).

396. **c** The payback period is the time required to recoup the cost of an investment. Mortgage refinancing analysis frequently uses the concept of payback period. Mortgage refinancing is considered when interest rates have dropped. Refinancing may require up-front interest payments and called points as well as a variety of administrative costs. In this example, the payback period is the time it takes for the savings in interest to equal the cost of the refinancing (Revoir and Davis 2016, 866).

397. **c** A formal code of ethics ensures that professionals understand and agree to uphold an ethical standard that puts the interests of the profession before their personal interests. Violation of the AHIMA Code of Ethics triggers a peer review process (Gordon and Gordon 2016, 915).

398. **b** Communication is key to engaging others in the vision and change process. The communication plan must offer groups the opportunity to talk back. Listening to staff concerns through the process is an important element (McClernon 2016, 948–949).

399. **c** The strategic goals and objectives need to be clearly outlined, with assignments for who will be accountable, timelines, allocation of resources, and measurements that will be used to ensure success of implementation. When a detailed implementation includes the elements laid out clearly—with timeframes and regular updates provided within the organization—the likelihood of strategic success increases significantly (McClernon 2016, 945)

400. **c** A process measure has a scientific basis for it. In this example, the percentage of antibiotics administered before surgery has been proven through evidence-based medicine, so it is scientifically based (Shaw and Carter 2015, 45).

401. **b** It is unfavorable and permanent because money that was not in the budget was spent on consulting services (Revoir and Davis 2016, 862).

402. **c** When the operating budget has been developed and approved, it is the responsibility of the department manager to ensure the budget goals are met and to explain all variances (Revoir and Davis 2016, 861).

403. **b** Quantity standards (also called productivity standards) and quality standards (also known as service standards) are generally used by managers to monitor individual employee performance and the performance of a functional unit or the department as a whole. To properly communicate performance standards, managers need to make the distinction between quantitative and qualitative standards and identify examples of each for the HIS functions. In the scenario, filing 50–60 records per hour is identifying the quantity of work rather than how well the work is being performed so it is a quantity standard (Oachs 2016, 800).

404. **d** The use of flowchart allows an individual to examine the process or procedure from all directions identifying bottlenecks or redundancies in a process. The technique makes it possible to gather the most important details so that everyone can understand the process and its contributing sub-processes in the same way (Shaw and Carter 2015, 198).

405. **d** Training is essential to the successful implementation of each new system. The implementation team must define who needs to be trained, who should do the training, how much training is required, and how the training will be accomplished (Biedermann and Dolezel 2017, 260).

406. **c** A mentor provides advice on developing skills and career options. In this situation Joan is mentoring Sandy towards her goal of becoming a privacy officer (Patena 2016, 761).

407. **a** A critical element of systems thinking is viewing an organization as an open system of interdependencies and connectedness rather than a collection of individual parts and professional enclaves. This approach sees interrelatedness as a whole and looks for patterns rather than snapshots of organizational activities and processes (Shaw and Carter 2015, 35).

408. **c** Conflict management focuses on working with the individuals involved to find a mutually acceptable solution. There are three ways to address conflict: compromise, control, and constructive confrontation (LeBlanc 2016, 744).

409. **b** The average turnaround time was calculated by dividing the total response days attributed to the volume of routine requests that were responded to within the reporting period by the volume of routine requests responded to. The calculation is: $(200 \times 3) + (100 \times 5) + (50 \times 8) + (50 \times 10) / 400 = 5$ days (Oachs 2016, 805).

410. **c** Serial work division is the consecutive handling of tasks or products by individuals who perform a specific function in sequence. Often referred to as a production line work division, serial work division tends to create task specialists (Oachs 2016, 791).

411. **a** To help all members understand the process, a team will undertake development of a flowchart. This work allows the team to thoroughly understand every step in the process and the sequence of steps. It provides a picture of each decision point and each event that must be completed. It readily points out places where there is redundancy and complex and problematic areas (Oachs 2016, 814).

412. **c** Strategic management is a process a leader uses for assessing a changing environment to create a vision of the future, determining how the organization fits into the anticipated environment based on its mission, vision, and knowledge of its strengths, weaknesses, opportunities, and threats, and then setting in motion a plan of action to position the organization accordingly (Oachs 2016, 928).

413. **b** Variances are often calculated on the monthly budget report. The organization's policies and procedures manual defines unacceptable variances or variances that must be explained. In identifying variances, it is important to recognize whether the variance is favorable or unfavorable and whether it is temporary or permanent (Revoir and Davis 2016, 862).

414. **a** An outcome measure may be the effect of care, treatment, or services on a customer (Shaw and Carter 2015, 46).

415. **c** Effective communication must occur at and between all levels of the organization from top leadership all the way to the front lines as well as with the persons working behind the scenes. Communication can take many forms these days including meetings, newsletters, and even social media (Biedermann and Dolezel 2017, 261).

416. **b** The capital budget looks at long-term investments. Such investments are usually related to improvements in the facility infrastructure, expansion of services, or replacement of existing assets. Capital investments focus on either the appropriateness of an investment (given the facility's investment guidelines) or choosing among different opportunities to invest. The capital budget is the facility's plan for allocating resources over and above the operating budget (Revoir and Davis 2016, 864).

417. **c** Qualitative standards specify the level of service quality expected from a function, such as accuracy rate. For example, assignment of diagnostic and procedure codes for inpatient records is at least 98 percent accurate (Revoir and Davis 2016, 799–800).

418. **b** Quantity standards (also called productivity standards) and quality standards (also known as service standards) are generally used by managers to monitor individual employee performance and the performance of a functional unit or the department as a whole. To properly communicate performance standards, managers need to make the distinction between quantitative and qualitative standards and identify examples of each for the HIS functions. In the scenario, completing five birth certificates per hour is identifying the quantity of work rather than how well the work is being performed so it is a quantity standard (Revoir and Davis 2016, 800).

419. **a** Standards that are measurable and relevant to an employee's overall performance are helpful in setting clear expectations. They also are useful in providing constructive feedback (LeBlanc 2016, 731).

420. **c** The rectangle with double lines on the side in a flowchart is a predefined process icon. This symbol represents the formal procedure that participants are expected to carry out the same way every time (Shaw and Carter 2015, 198).

421. **c** Liquidity refers to the ease with which assets can be turned into cash. This is important because payroll, loan payments, and other financial obligations are typically paid in cash (Revoir and Davis 2016, 852).

422. **a** Empowerment is the concept of providing employees with the tools and resources to solve problems themselves. In other words, employees obtain power over their work situation by assuming responsibility. Empowered employees have the freedom to contribute ideas and perform their jobs in the best possible way (Patena 2016, 779).

423. **a** A contract action arises when one party claims that the other party has failed to meet an obligation set forth in a valid contract. Another way to state this is that the other party has breached the contract. The resolution available is either compensation or performance of the obligation (Rinehart-Thompson 2016, 56).

424. **c** In-service education is a continuous process that builds on the basic skills learned through new employee orientation and on-the-job training. It is concerned with teaching employees specific skills and behaviors required to maintain job performance (Patena 2016, 762).

425. **c** There are several laws that affect discrimination in employment on the basis of race, color, religion, age, sex, national origin, citizenship status, and veterans status. Most organizations would like to hire someone whose vision for the organization is in line with their own vision (Reynolds and Brodnik 2017c, 490)

426. **b** Internal procedures to reduce risk of groupthink include brainstorming, revisiting important decisions, monitoring the degree of consensus and disagreement, rotating the devil's advocate role, and actively seeking contradictory information. External procedures include discussing decisions with outside experts and nonteam members and inviting external observers to provide feedback on meetings, decisions, and team processes. Such procedures increase awareness of group processes and enhance skills at arriving at better decisions (Swenson 2016, 686–687).

427. **d** Alternative staffing structures offer flexibility in hours, location, and job responsibilities as a method to attract and retain employees and eliminate staffing shortages. Some examples are job sharing, outsourcing, flextime, and telecommuting (Oachs 2016, 795).

428. **b** The Americans with Disabilities Act of 1990 protects individuals with disabilities. Employees must be able to perform the necessary functions of a job with "reasonable accommodations," which include modifications to the workplace or conditions of employment so that a disabled worker can perform the job (Reynolds and Brodnik 2017c, 492).

429. **b** A project differs from the day-to-day operations of an organization. Operations are concerned with the everyday jobs needed to run the business. The personnel involved in the operational aspects of the business perform the same functions on a routine basis. This work does not end. In contrast, a project has a precise, expected result produced by defined resources within a specific time frame (Olson 2016, 875).

430. **d** Zero-based budgets apply to organizations for which each budget cycle poses the opportunity to continue or discontinue services based on the availability of resources. Every department or activity must be justified and prioritized annually in order to effectively allocate the organization's resources. Professional associations and charitable foundations, for example, routinely use zero-based budgeting (AHIMA 2014, 46).

431. **b** A project plan starts with a work breakdown structure (WBS), or task list. The WBS is a hierarchical list of steps needed to complete the project. This structure provides levels that are similar to the concept of a book outline. Each level drills down to more detail. The lowest level is the task level, which is the level to which resources are assigned and work effort estimates are made (Olson 2016, 899; Oachs and Watters 2016, 1040).

432. **d** Deliverables are a tangible output produced by the completion of project tasks (Olson 2016, 899).

433. **d** Ethical obligations to the public include advocating change when patterns or system problems are not in the best interest of the patients, such as reporting violations of practice standards to the proper authorities (Gordon and Gordon 2016, 917).

434. **a** The arithmetic difference between total revenue and total expenses is net income (Revoir and Davis 2016, 849).

435. **d** The symbol is called the manual input icon in flowcharting. This symbol represents points in the flowchart description of the process where the participants must record data in paper- or computer-based formats (Shaw and Carter 2015, 200).

436. **d** Strategic management is a process a leader uses for assessing a changing environment to create a vision of the future, determining how the organization fits into the anticipated environment based on its mission, vision, and knowledge of its strengths, weaknesses, opportunities, and threats, and then setting in motion a plan of action to position the organization accordingly (Gordon and Gordon 2016, 928).

437. **b** Each licensed independent contractor or practitioner who provides care under the auspices of a healthcare organization must do so in accordance with delineated clinical privileges. One of the requirements for these privileges is for the individual to carry his or her own professional liability insurance and therefore that practitioner is considered an independent contractor within the healthcare organization (Shaw and Carter 2015, 345).

438. **d** An income statement summarizes the organization's revenue and expense transactions during the fiscal year. The income statement can be prepared at any point in time and reflects results up to that point. The income statement contains only income and expense accounts and reflects only the activity for the current fiscal year (Revoir and Davis 2016, 849).

439. **b** A balance sheet is a snapshot of the accounting equation at a point in time (Revoir and Davis 2016, 849).

440. **a** Recruitment is the process of finding, soliciting, and attracting new employees. However, the manager should be sure to understand the organization's recruitment and hiring policies and to seek the assistance of the HR department before the vacancy is publicized (LeBlanc 2016, 732).

441. **c** Strategic managers develop skills reflecting the implications and opportunities afforded by trends. Whether reading a journal or discussing new ideas with others, strategic managers are always testing new ideas, identifying those that have merit, and discarding those that do not. They are creating links between the trends and the value-adding actions they can take (McClernon 2016, 930).

442. **c** The early majority comprises about 34 percent of the organization. Although usually not leaders, the individuals in this group represent the backbone of the organization, are deliberate in thinking and acceptance of an idea, and serve as a natural bridge between early and late adopters (Swenson 2016, 701).

443. **d** Adults like feedback on their performance. It is important to understand the concept of the learning curve. When a new task is learned, productivity may decrease while a great deal of material is actually being learned. Later, there is little new learning, but productivity may increase greatly. Either situation can be frustrating, so guidance and feedback are important to help employees understand what they have accomplished (Patena 2016, 769).

444. **b** The needs analysis is critical to the design of the training plan. This approach typically focuses on three levels: the organization, the specific job tasks, and the individual employee (Patena 2016, 753).

445. **b** All contracts include representations or warranties of some sort, which are statements of facts existing at the time the contract is made. These statements are made by one party to induce the other party to enter the contract. Typically, these statements relate to the quality of goods or services purchased or leased (Klaver 2017b, 129–130).

446. **a** Blended learning uses several delivery methods thereby gaining the advantages and reducing the disadvantages of each method alone (Patena 2016, 772).

447. **d** HIM professionals must factor several criteria into their decision making. Ethicists provide assistance in this process. When faced with an ethical issue, the HIM professional should evaluate the ethical problem following these steps: what are the facts; who are the stakeholders; what are the options; what is the decision; what justifies the choice, and what is the prevention. When a decision must be made about an issue and not identified following the steps, the decision most likely will be based on an individual's narrow moral perspective of right or wrong (Gordon and Gordon 2016, 919).

448. **b** A strategy map is a tool that provides a visual representation of an organization's critical objectives and the relationships among them that drive organizational performance. Depicting change as a road map is a useful way to help others understand the goals and the course of change (McClernon 2016, 951).

449. **c** Cost–benefit feasibility is used to determine if an EHR initiative is appropriate for the organization at this time; it measures the costs associated with acquisition of hardware and software, installation, implementation, and ongoing maintenance (Amatayakul 2016, 104–105).

450. **c** A Gantt chart is used to illustrate project tasks, phases, and milestones and their start, end, and completion dates. It helps to show where more than one task must be performed simultaneously. The column labeled D is showing the progress of the task "1.1 Write test scenario" (Malmgren and Solberg 2016, 243).

451. **b** Through the system implementation, stakeholders should be kept apprised of the project status. This is important to ensure the various users begin to understand the project and do not get the feeling that it is happening in a vacuum. Communication can be accomplished through formal and informal methods. Communication between stakeholders and standards setting organizations would not occur during system implementation (Biedermann and Dolezel 2017, 261).

452. **b** Quantity standards (also called productivity standards) and quality standards (also known as service standards) are generally used by managers to monitor individual employee performance and the performance of a functional unit or the department as a whole. To properly communicate performance standards, managers need to make the distinction between quantitative and qualitative standards and identify examples of each for the HIS functions. In the scenario, transcribing 1,500 lines per day is identifying the quantity of work rather than how well the work is being performed so it is a quantity standard (Oachs 2016, 800).

453. **c** In cross-training, the employee learns to perform the jobs of many team members. This method is most useful when work teams are involved (Patena 2016, 761).

454. **d** Flextime generally refers to the employee's ability to work by varying his or her starting and stopping hours around a core of midshift hours, such as 10 a.m. to 1 p.m. Depending on their position and the institution, employees may have a certain degree of freedom in determining their hours (Oachs 2016, 795).

455. **a** The strategic profile identifies the existing key services or products of the department or organization, the nature of its customers and users, the nature of its market segments, and the nature of its geographic markets (McClernon 2016, 934; Robert 2006, 53–542).

456. **a** The purpose of hold harmless or indemnification clauses is to either transfer or assume liability. For example, the indemnitor (party assuming liability) may agree to hold the other party harmless against claims arising from the indemnitor's own actions or failures to act. This means if actions (or inactions) result in harm to the other party, the indemnitor will seek to make that party whole, often through some sort of compensation (Klaver 2017b, 129–130).

457. **d** To develop an orientation program, it is helpful to begin with a task analysis to determine the specific skills required for the job. The job description and the job specification are excellent sources for this part of the process. A task analysis is part of the needs assessment (Patena 2016, 753).

458. **a** Appointments to the board of directors is important information, but the Joint Commission requires detailed information on the responsibilities and actions of the board, not necessarily its composition. The Joint Commission requires healthcare organizations to collect data on each of these areas: medication management, blood and blood product use, restraint and seclusion use, behavior management and treatment, operative and other invasive procedures, and resuscitation and its outcomes (Shaw and Carter 2015, 378, 382).

459. **d** Sometimes problems arise because of conflicts among employees. It is common for people to disagree, and sometimes a difference of opinion can increase creativity. However, too much conflict can also waste time, reduce productivity, and decrease morale. When taken to the extreme, it can threaten the safety of employees and cause damage to property (LeBlanc 2016, 744).

460. **c** Work sampling is a technique of work measurement that involves using statistical probability (determined through random sample observations) to characterize the performance of the department and its work (functional) units (Oachs 2016, 803).

RESOURCES

References

Primary References

American Health Information Management Association. 2014. *Pocket Glossary of Health Information Management and Technology,* 4th ed. Chicago: American Health Information Management Association.

Amatayakul, M.K. 2017. *Electronic Health Records: A Practical Guide for Professionals and Organizations,* 6th ed. Chicago: American Health Information Management Association.

Amatayakul, M.K. 2016. Health Information Systems Strategic Planning. Chapter 13 in *Health Information Management: Concepts, Principles, and Practice,* 5th ed. Edited by P. Oachs and A. Watters. Chicago: American Health Information Management Association.

Biedermann, S. and D. Dolezel. 2017. *Introduction to Healthcare Informatics,* 2nd ed. Chicago: American Health Information Management Association.

Bowman, S. 2017. Corporate Compliance. Chapter 18 in *Fundamentals of Law for Health Informatics and Information Management*, 3rd ed. Edited by M.S. Brodnik, L.A. Rinehart-Thompson, and R.B. Reynolds. Chicago: American Health Information Management Association.

Brinda, D. and A.L. Watters. 2016. Data Privacy, Confidentiality, and Security. Chapter 11 in *Health Information Management: Concepts, Principles, and Practice,* 5th ed. Edited by P. Oachs and A. Watters. Chicago: American Health Information Management Association.

Brodnik, M.S. 2017a. Introduction to the Fundamentals of Law for Health Informatics and Information Management. Chapter 1 in *Fundamentals of Law for Health Informatics and Information Management*, 3rd ed. Edited by M.S. Brodnik, L.A. Rinehart-Thompson, and R.B. Reynolds. Chicago: American Health Information Management Association.

Brodnik, M.S. 2017b. Access, Use, and Disclosure and Release of Health Information. Chapter 15 in *Fundamentals of Law for Health Informatics and Information Management*, 3rd ed. Edited by M.S. Brodnik, L.A. Rinehart-Thompson, and R.B. Reynolds. Chicago: American Health Information Management Association.

Brodnik, M.S. 2017c. Required Reporting and Mandatory Disclosure Laws. Chapter 16 in *Fundamentals of Law for Health Informatics and Information Management*, 3rd ed. Edited by M.S. Brodnik, L.A. Rinehart-Thompson, and R.B. Reynolds. Chicago: American Health Information Management Association.

Brodnik, M.S. and R.B. Reynolds. 2017. Risk Management, Quality Improvement, and Patient Safety. Chapter 17 in *Fundamentals of Law for Health Informatics and Information Management*, 3rd ed. Edited by M.S. Brodnik, L.A. Rinehart-Thompson, and R.B. Reynolds. Chicago: American Health Information Management Association.

Brodnik, M.S., L.A. Rinehart-Thompson, and R.B. Reynolds. 2017. *Fundamentals of Law for Health Informatics and Information Management*, 3rd ed. Chicago: American Health Information Management Association.

Casto, A.B. and E. Forrestal. 2015. *Principles of Healthcare Reimbursement,* 5th ed. Chicago: American Health Information Management Association.

Edgerton, C.G. 2016. Healthcare Statistics. Chapter 16 in *Health Information Management: Concepts, Principles, and Practice,* 5th ed. Edited by P. Oachs and A. Watters. Chicago: American Health Information Management Association.

Fahrenholz, C.G. 2013a. Clinical Documentation and the Health Record. Chapter 2 in *Documentation for Health Records*. Edited by C. G. Fahrenholz and R. Russo. Chicago: American Health Information Management Association.

Fahrenholz, C.G. 2013b. Principal and Ancillary Functions of the Healthcare Record. Chapter 3 in *Documentation for Health Records*. Edited by C. G. Fahrenholz and R. Russo. Chicago: American Health Information Management Association.

Fahrenholz, C.G. 2013c. Documentation for Statistical Reporting and Public Health. Chapter 4 in *Documentation for Health Records*. Edited by C. G. Fahrenholz and R. Russo. Chicago: American Health Information Management Association.

Fahrenholz, C.G. 2013d. Healthcare Delivery. Chapter 1 in *Documentation for Health Records*. Edited by C. G. Fahrenholz and R. Russo. Chicago: American Health Information Management Association.

Fahrenholz, C.G. and R. Russo, eds. 2013. *Documentation for Health Records*. Chicago: American Health Information Management Association.

Forrestal, E. 2016. Research Methods. Chapter 19 in *Health Information Management: Concepts, Principles, and Practice,* 5th ed. Edited by P. Oachs and A. Watters. Chicago: American Health Information Management Association.

Fuller, S.R. 2016. The US Healthcare Delivery System. Chapter 1 in *Health Information Management: Concepts, Principles, and Practice,* 5th ed. Edited by P. Oachs and A. Watters. Chicago: American Health Information Management Association.

Giannangelo, K. 2015. *Healthcare Code Sets, Clinical Terminologies, and Classification Systems,* 3rd ed. Chicago: American Health Information Management Association.

Giannangelo, K. 2016. Clinical Terminologies, Classifications, and Code Systems. Chapter 5 in *Health Information Management: Concepts, Principles, and Practice,* 5th ed. Edited by P. Oachs and A. Watters. Chicago: American Health Information Management Association.

Gordon, M.L. and L.L. Gordon. 2016. Ethical Issues in Health Information. Chapter 28 in *Health Information Management: Concepts, Principles, and Practice,* 5th ed. Edited by P. Oachs and A. Watters. Chicago: American Health Information Management Association.

Hazelwood, A.C. and C.A. Venable. 2016. Reimbursement Methodologies. Chapter 7 in *Health Information Management: Concepts, Principles, and Practice,* 5th ed. Edited by P. Oachs and A. Watters. Chicago: American Health Information Management Association.

Hess, P. 2015. *Clinical Documentation Improvement: Principles and Practice*. Chicago: American Health Information Management Association.

Horton, L.A. 2016. *Calculating and Reporting Healthcare Statistics,* 5th ed. Chicago: American Health Information Management Association.

Hunt, T.J. 2016. Clinical Documentation Improvement and Coding Compliance. Chapter 9 in *Health Information Management: Concepts, Principles, and Practice,* 5th ed. Edited by P. Oachs and A. Watters. Chicago: American Health Information Management Association.

James, E.L. 2013a. Long-Term Care Hospitals. Chapter 10 in *Documentation for Health Records*. Edited by C. G. Fahrenholz and R. Russo. Chicago: American Health Information Management Association.

James, E.L. 2013b. Facility-Based Long-Term Care. Chapter 11 in *Documentation for Health Records*. Edited by C. G. Fahrenholz and R. Russo. Chicago: American Health Information Management Association.

James, E.L. 2013c. Federal and State Requirements and Accreditation Guidelines. Chapter 8 in *Documentation for Health Records*. Edited by C. G. Fahrenholz and R. Russo. Chicago: American Health Information Management Association.

Johns, M. 2015. *Enterprise Health Information Management and Data Governance*. Chicago: American Health Information Management Association.

Johns, M. 2016. Data Governance and Stewardship. Chapter 3 in *Health Information Management: Concepts, Principles, and Practice,* 5th ed. Edited by P. Oachs and A. Watters. Chicago: American Health Information Management Association.

Kelly, J. and P. Greenstone. 2016. *Management of the Health Information Professional*. Chicago: American Health Information Management Association.

Klaver, J.C. 2017a. Evidence. Chapter 5 in *Fundamentals of Law for Health Informatics and Information Management*, 3rd ed. Edited by M.S. Brodnik, L.A. Rinehart-Thompson, and R.B. Reynolds. Chicago: American Health Information Management Association.

Klaver, J.C. 2017b. Corporations, Contracts, and Antitrust Legal Issues. Chapter 7 in *Fundamentals of Law for Health Informatics and Information Management*, 3rd ed. Edited by M.S. Brodnik, L.A. Rinehart-Thompson, and R.B. Reynolds. Chicago: American Health Information Management Association.

Klaver, J.C. 2017c. Consent to Treatment. Chapter 8 in *Fundamentals of Law for Health Informatics and Information Management*, 3rd ed. Edited by M.S. Brodnik, L.A. Rinehart-Thompson, and R.B. Reynolds. Chicago: American Health Information Management Association.

Kuehn, L. 2017. *Procedural Coding and Reimbursement for Physician Services: Applying Current Procedural Terminology and HCPCS 2017*. Chicago: American Health Information Management Association.

Kuehn, L.M. and T.M. Jorwic. 2017. ICD-10-PCS *An Applied Approach 2017*. Chicago: American Health Information Management Association.

Malmgren, C. and C.J. Solberg 2016. Revenue Cycle Management. Chapter 8 in *Health Information Management: Concepts, Principles, and Practice,* 5th ed. Edited by P. Oachs and A. Watters. Chicago: American Health Information Management Association.

Marc, D. 2016. Data Visualization. Chapter 18 in *Health Information Management: Concepts, Principles, and Practice,* 5th ed. Edited by P. Oachs and A. Watters. Chicago: American Health Information Management Association.

Marc, D. and R. Sandefer. 2016. *Data Analytics in Healthcare Research: Tools and Strategies*. Chicago: American Health Information Management Association.

McCann, P. 2016. Health Information Exchange. Chapter 15 in *Health Information Management: Concepts, Principles, and Practice,* 5th ed. Edited by P. Oachs and A. Watters. Chicago: American Health Information Management Association.

McClernon, S.E. 2016. Strategic Thinking and Management. Chapter 29 in *Health Information Management: Concepts, Principles, and Practice,* 5th ed. Edited by P. Oachs and A. Watters. Chicago: American Health Information Management Association.

Munn, K.M. 2013. Behavioral Healthcare. Chapter 13 in *Documentation for Health Records*. Edited by C. G. Fahrenholz and R. Russo. Chicago: American Health Information Management Association.

LeBlanc, M.M. 2016. Human Resource Management. Chapter 23 in *Health Information Management: Concepts, Principles, and Practice,* 5th ed. Edited by P. Oachs and A. Watters. Chicago: American Health Information Management Association.

Oachs, P.K. 2016. Work Design and Process Improvement. Chapter 25 in *Health Information Management: Concepts, Principles, and Practice,* 5th ed. Edited by P. Oachs and A. Watters. Chicago: American Health Information Management Association.

Oachs, P.K. and A.L. Watters, eds. 2016. *Health Information Management: Concepts, Principles, and Practice,* 5th ed. Chicago: American Health Information Management Association.

Olenik, K. and R.B. Reynolds. 2017. Security Threats and Controls. Chapter 13 in *Fundamentals of Law for Health Informatics and Information Management*, 3rd ed. Edited by M.S. Brodnik, L.A. Rinehart-Thompson, and R.B. Reynolds. Chicago: American Health Information Management Association.

Olson, B.D. 2016. Project Management. Chapter 27 in *Health Information Management: Concepts, Principles, and Practice,* 5th ed. Edited by P. Oachs and A. Watters. Chicago: American Health Information Management Association.

Palkie, B. 2016a. Clinical Classifications, Vocabularies, Terminologies, and Standards. Chapter 5 in *Health Information Management: Concepts, Principles, and Practice*, 5th ed. Edited by P. Oachs and A. Watters. Chicago: American Health Information Management Association.

Palkie, B. 2016b. Organizational Compliance and Risk. Chapter 10 in *Health Information Management: Concepts, Principles, and Practice,* 5th ed. Edited by P. Oachs and A. Watters. Chicago: American Health Information Management Association.

Patena, K.R. 2016. Employee Training and Development. Chapter 24 in *Health Information Management: Concepts, Principles, and Practice,* 5th ed. Edited by P. Oachs and A. Watters. Chicago: American Health Information Management Association.

Revoir, R. and N. Davis. 2016. Financial Management. Chapter 26 in *Health Information Management: Concepts, Principles, and Practice,* 5th ed. Edited by P. Oachs and A. Watters. Chicago: American Health Information Management Association.

Reynolds, R.B. and M.S. Brodnik. 2017a. The HIPAA Security Rule. Chapter 12 in *Fundamentals of Law for Health Informatics and Information Management*, 3rd ed. Edited by M.S. Brodnik, L.A. Rinehart-Thompson, and R.B. Reynolds. Chicago: American Health Information Management Association.

Reynolds, R.B. and M.S. Brodnik. 2017b. Medical Staff. Chapter 19 in *Fundamentals of Law for Health Informatics and Information Management*, 3rd ed. Edited by M.S. Brodnik, L.A. Rinehart-Thompson, and R.B. Reynolds. Chicago: American Health Information Management Association.

Reynolds, R.B. and M.S. Brodnik. 2017c. Workplace Law. Chapter 20 in *Fundamentals of Law for Health Informatics and Information Management*, 3rd ed. Edited by M.S. Brodnik, L.A. Rinehart-Thompson, and R.B. Reynolds. Chicago: American Health Information Management Association.

Reynolds, R.B. and M. Sharp. 2016. Heath Record Content and Documentation. Chapter 4 in *Health Information Management: Concepts, Principles, and Practice,* 5th ed. Edited by P. Oachs and A. Watters. Chicago: American Health Information Management Association.

Rinehart-Thompson, L.A. 2017a. Legal Proceedings. Chapter 4 in *Fundamentals of Law for Health Informatics and Information Management*, 3rd ed. Edited by M.S. Brodnik, L.A. Rinehart-Thompson, and R.B. Reynolds. Chicago: American Health Information Management Association.

Rinehart-Thompson, L.A. 2017b. Tort Law. Chapter 6 in *Fundamentals of Law for Health Informatics and Information Management*, 3rd ed. Edited by M.S. Brodnik, L.A. Rinehart-Thompson, and R.B. Reynolds. Chicago: American Health Information Management Association.

Rinehart-Thompson, L.A. 2017c. Legal Health Record: Maintenance, Content, Documentation, and Disposition. Chapter 9 in *Fundamentals of Law for Health Informatics and Information Management*, 3rd ed. Edited by M.S. Brodnik, L.A. Rinehart-Thompson, and R.B. Reynolds. Chicago: American Health Information Management Association.

Rinehart-Thompson, L.A. 2017d. HIPAA Privacy Rule: Part I. Chapter 10 in *Fundamentals of Law for Health Informatics and Information Management*, 3rd ed. Edited by M.S. Brodnik, L.A. Rinehart-Thompson, and R.B. Reynolds. Chicago: American Health Information Management Association.

Rinehart-Thompson, L.A. 2017e. HIPAA Privacy Rule: Part II. Chapter 11 in *Fundamentals of Law for Health Informatics and Information Management*, 3rd ed. Edited by M.S. Brodnik, L.A. Rinehart-Thompson, and R.B. Reynolds. Chicago: American Health Information Management Association.

Rinehart-Thompson, L.A. 2016. Legal Issues in Health Information Management. Chapter 2 in *Health Information Management: Concepts, Principles, and Practice,* 5th ed. Edited by P. Oachs and A. Watters. Chicago: American Health Information Management Association.

Rinehart-Thompson, L.A. 2013. *Introduction to Health Information Privacy and Security*. Chicago: American Health Information Management Association.

Rossiter, S. 2013. Health Records in Ambulatory Care. Chapter 9 in *Documentation for Health Records*. Edited by C. G. Fahrenholz and R. Russo. Chicago: American Health Information Management Association.

Russo, R. 2013a. Clinical Information and Nonclinical Data. Chapter 5 in *Documentation for Health Records*. Edited by C. G. Fahrenholz and R. Russo. Chicago: American Health Information Management Association.

Russo, R. 2013b. Health Record Design. Chapter 6 in *Documentation for Health Records*. Edited by C. G. Fahrenholz and R. Russo. Chicago: American Health Information Management Association.

Russo, R. 2013c. Best Practices in Health Record Documentation. Chapter 7 in *Documentation for Health Records*. Edited by C. G. Fahrenholz and R. Russo. Chicago: American Health Information Management Association.

Sandefer, R.H. 2016a. Health Information Technologies. Chapter 12 in *Health Information Management: Concepts, Principles, and Practice,* 5th ed. Edited by P. Oachs and A. Watters. Chicago: American Health Information Management Association.

Sandefer, R.H. 2016b. Consumer Health Informatics. Chapter 14 in *Health Information Management: Concepts, Principles, and Practice,* 5th ed. Edited by P. Oachs and A. Watters. Chicago: American Health Information Management Association.

Sayles, N.B. and K.C. Trawick. 2014. *Introduction to Computer Systems for Health Information Technology,* 2nd ed. Chicago: American Health Information Management Association.

Schraffenberger, L.A. and L. Kuehn. 2011. *Effective Management of Coding Services,* 3rd ed. Chicago: American Health Information Management Association.

Schraffenberger, L.A. and B. Palkie. 2017. *Basic ICD-10-CM and ICD-10-PCS Coding 2017*. Chicago: American Health Information Management Association.

Sharp, M.Y. and C. Madlock-Brown. 2016. Data Management. Chapter 6 in *Health Information Management: Concepts, Principles, and Practice,* 5th ed. Edited by P. Oachs and A. Watters. Chicago: American Health Information Management Association.

Shaw, P.L. and D. Carter. 2015. *Quality and Performance Improvement in Healthcare: Theory, Practice, and Management*, 6th ed. Chicago: American Health Information Management Association.

Swenson, D.X. 2016. Managing and Leading During Organizational Change. Chapter 22 in *Health Information Management: Concepts, Principles, and Practice,* 5th ed. Edited by P. Oachs and A. Watters. Chicago: American Health Information Management Association.

Theodos, K. 2017. Law and Ethics. Chapter 2 in *Fundamentals of Law for Health Informatics and Information Management*, 3rd ed. Edited by M.S. Brodnik, L.A. Rinehart-Thompson, and R.B. Reynolds. Chicago: American Health Information Management Association.

Thomason, M.C. 2013. *HIPAA by Example: Application of Privacy Laws,* 2nd ed. Chicago: American Health Information Management Association.

Watzlaf, V.J.M. 2016. Biomedical and Research Support. Chapter 20 in *Health Information Management: Concepts, Principles, and Practice,* 5th ed. Edited by P. Oachs and A. Watters. Chicago: American Health Information Management Association.

White, M.J. 2013. Home Care and Hospice Documentation, Accreditation, Liability, and Standards. Chapter 12 in *Documentation for Health Records*. Edited by C. G. Fahrenholz and R. Russo. Chicago: American Health Information Management Association.

White, S. 2016a. *A Practical Approach to Analyzing Healthcare Data,* 3rd ed. Chicago: American Health Information Management Association.

White, S. 2016b. Healthcare Data Analytics. Chapter 17 in *Health Information Management: Concepts, Principles, and Practice,* 5th ed. Edited by P. Oachs and A. Watters. Chicago: American Health Information Management Association.

Wilson, D.D. 2010. *Responding to a Recovery Audit Contractor (RAC) Evaluation*. Chicago: American Health Information Management Association.

Secondary References from Answer Key Rationales

45 CFR 160:103: General administrative requirements: General Provisions: Definitions. 2006.

45 CFR 164: 501: Uses and disclosures of protected health information (general rules). 2006.

45 CFR 164: 502b: Minimum necessary. 2006.

45 CFR 164: 506: Uses and disclosures for which authorization is required. 2006.

45 CFR 164: 508: Uses and disclosures for which authorization is required. 2006.

45 CFR 164: 514: Uses and disclosures of protected health information (general rules). 2006.

American Health Information Management Association. 2013 (January 25). Analysis of Modifications to the HIPAA Privacy, Security, Enforcement, and Breach Notification Rules under the Health Information Technology for Economic and Clinical Health Act and the Genetic Information Nondiscrimination Act; Other Modifications to the HIPAA Rules. http://bok.ahima.org/PdfView?oid=106127.

American Health Information Management Association. 2011. Fundamentals of the Legal Health Record and Designated Record Set. *Journal of AHIMA*. 82(2). http://bok.ahima.org/doc?oid=104008#.VuhZEvkrK9I.

American Health Information Management Association. 2010 (August). Overview of the Proposed Rule: Modifications to the HIPAA Privacy, Security, and Enforcement Rules Under the Health Information Technology for Economic and Clinical Health Act. http://bok.ahima.org/PdfView?oid=106287.

American Health Information Management Association. 2009 (March). Analysis of Health Care Confidentiality, Privacy, and Security Provisions of the American Recovery and Reinvestment Act of 2009, Public Law 111-5. Chicago: American Health Information Management Association. http://bok.ahima.org/PdfView?oid=91955.

American Health Information Management Association. 2009 (February). Redisclosure of Patient Health Information (Updated). *Journal of AHIMA*. 80(2):51–54.

American Medical Informatics Association. 2015. Consumer Health Informatics. https://www.amia.org/applications-informatics/consumer-health-informatics.

American Recovery and Reinvestment Act of 2009. Title XIII: Health Information Technology. Subtitle D: Privacy. Part 1: Improved Privacy Provisions and Security Provisions, Sections 13401–13411.

Center for Medicare and Medicaid Services (CMS). 2010. *CMS's RAI Version 3.0 Manual: Medicare Skilled Nursing Facility Prospective Payment System (SNF PPS)*. http://www.cms.gov/SNFPPS/.

Office for Civil Rights, Department of Health and Human Services. 2012. *Guidance Regarding Methods for De-identification of Protected Health Information in accordance with the Health Insurance Portability and Accountability Act (HIPAA) Privacy Rule*. http://www.hhs.gov/ocr/privacy/hipaa/understanding/coveridentities/De-identification/hhs_deid_guidance.pdf.

Pozgar, G.D. 2012. *Legal Aspects of Health Care Administration,* 11th ed. Sudbury, MA: Jones and Bartlett Learning.

Rob, P. and C. Coronel. 2009. *Database Systems: Design, Implementation, and Management,* 8th ed. Boston, MA: Course Technology, Thomson Learning.

Robert, M. 2006. *The New Strategic Thinking: Pure and Simple*. New York: McGraw-Hill.

U.S. Department of Health and Human Services. 2012. Health Information Privacy. Breaches Affecting 500 or More Individuals. http://www.hhs.gov/ocr/privacy/hipaa/administrative/breachnotificationrule/breachtool.html.

Hospital Statistical Formulas Used for the RHIA Exam

Hospital Statistical Formulas Used for the RHIA Exam

Average Daily Census

$$\frac{\text{Total service days for the unit for the period}}{\text{Total number of days in the period}}$$

Average Length of Stay

$$\frac{\text{Total length of stay (discharge days)}}{\text{Total discharges (includes deaths)}}$$

Percentage of Occupancy

$$\frac{\text{Total service days for a period}}{\text{Total bed count days in the period}} \times 100$$

Hospital Death Rate (Gross)

$$\frac{\text{Number of deaths of inpatients in period}}{\text{Number of discharges (including deaths)}} \times 100$$

Gross Autopsy Rate

$$\frac{\text{Total inpatient autopsies for a given period}}{\text{Total inpatient deaths for the period}} \times 100$$

Net Autopsy Rate

$$\frac{\text{Total inpatients for a given period}}{\text{Total inpatient deaths} - \text{unautopsied coroners' or medical examiners' cases}} \times 100$$

Hospital Autopsy Rate (Adjusted)

$$\frac{\text{Total hospital autopsies}}{\text{Number of deaths of hospital patients whose bodies are available for hospital autopsy}} \times 100$$

Fetal Death Rate

$$\frac{\text{Total number of intermediate and/or late fetal deaths for a period}}{\text{Total number of live births} + \text{intermediate and late fetal deaths for the period}} \times 100$$

Neonatal Mortality Rate (Death Rate)

$$\frac{\text{Total number of newborn deaths for a period}}{\text{Total number of newborn infant discharges (including deaths) for the period}} \times 100$$

Maternal Mortality Rate (Death Rate)

$$\frac{\text{Total number of direct maternal deaths for a period}}{\text{Total number of obstetrical discharges (including deaths) for the period}} \times 100$$

Caesarean-Section Rate

$$\frac{\text{Total number of caesarean sections performed in a period}}{\text{Total number of deliveries in the period (including caesarean sections)}} \times 100$$